RIGHT BODY FOR YOU

RIGHT BODY FOR YOU

By Gary M. Douglas

ACCESS CONSCIOUSNESS®
PUBLISHING

Right Body for You

ISBN: 978-1-939261-19-9

The author and publisher of the book do not make any claim or guarantee for any physical, mental, emotional, spiritual, or financial result. All products, services and information provided by the author are for general education and entertainment purposes only. The information provided herein is in no way a substitute for medical advice. In the event you use any of the information contained in this book for yourself, the author and publisher assume no responsibility for your actions.

Published by Access Consciousness® Publishing

Printed in the United States of America

Contents

Right Body for You is about recognizing how you are creating your body. It's about discovering whether you have the body that your body wants to be—and what you need to do to create the body your body wishes to be.

Everything we teach in Access Consciousness™ is about giving you tools, techniques, and systems that will unlock whatever is limiting you. I'm a pragmatist. As long as something works, I keep using it. When it stops working, I do something different. If something doesn't work for you, don't do it.

Part One

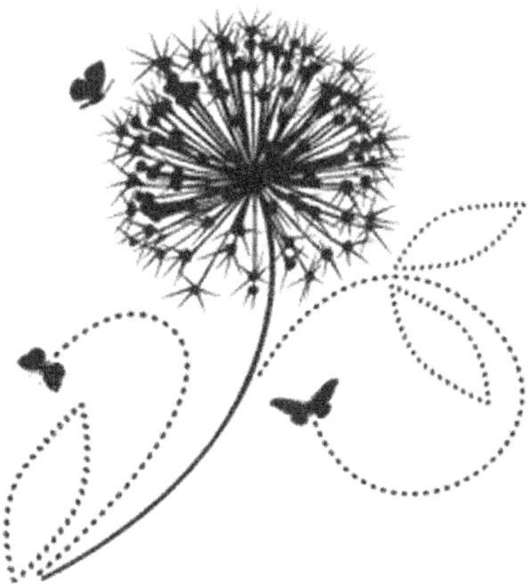

by Donnielle Carter

Chapter 1

From Size 16 To Size 6 In Four Months

When you begin to listen to your body, something entirely different can show up.

Donnielle Carter is a vibrant woman with reddish hair and warm brown eyes. She loves to wear silky clothes that show off her curves. She talks freely, laughs often, and enjoys being in the limelight. She is an Access Consciousness facilitator and a radio show host with many years of experience in radio and TV broadcasting.

Several years ago, Donnielle, who is five foot two inches tall, wore a size 18. Her loose jeans were size 20. When she completed her first Access class, she was wearing a size 16. Four months later, she was wearing a size 6. I have asked her to share the story of how she used Access processes to go from a size 16 to a size 6 in four months.

~ Gary M. Douglas

I graduated from Brigham Young University with a degree in broadcast production, and I worked for many years as the promotions manager for a major TV station. Everything that was on-air outside of programming was my responsibility. I was in charge of promotional events and contests, and I designed radio ads, billboards, Web content, even stationery and business cards. I came up through the production side of things, so I would also edit video and have won some awards for my video editing. I also did audio editing, camera work, shot cameras, microphones, have done location shoots, and more.

Because I worked in promotions, I often had to be in front of people. We did events, we were at expos, and we sponsored premieres and that kind of thing. We often had big contests to give away tickets for the premieres of movies. Before the movie started, it would be my job to stand in front of the movie theater crowd and say, "Hey! Thanks for coming out. We welcome you!"

Staying Hidden

I hated it when I had to publicly represent the station because I knew I was fat, I felt ugly, and I was going to be judged. I'm Five foot two inches tall, and I wore a size 18. My loose jeans were a size 20. I wasn't happy with myself, obviously, and I couldn't bear the thought that people were going to look at me and judge me. I would often pay—or bribe—someone from the station to get up in front of the audience and talk for me. I was protecting the station in some warped way. I felt I didn't represent them well because of the way I looked.

I did whatever I could do to remain hidden, and I would go to any lengths to avoid being on camera. I would climb over boxes or cables to get around any camera, even if I knew it wasn't turned on. My desire to remain out of sight made it hard for me to do my job—because when you're in promotions, you're in the public eye.

I spent a lot of time in a fantasy world where I was a different person. I'd be skinny and pretty and attractive. I'd have fantasy boyfriends, and I'd do fun things with fantasy friends. I would become just present enough to talk to people and get my work done—then I'd go back into my fantasy world. I recently found some pictures of me from that time and showed them to my mom. She looked at the pictures and said, "I just didn't see how big you had gotten. How could I have not seen that? I thought you were fine."

But I knew I wasn't fine. My mom is a nutritionist. I didn't want her to introduce me to people as her daughter, because I didn't want her friends to say, "Look at your fat daughter. She's obviously unhealthy." I knew I was unhealthy, I knew I was toxic, but I chose to ignore it and pretend it wasn't there.

My mom was interested in everything that came across her path—metaphysics, homeopathy, naturopathy. She read alot and went to classes. She had a radio show where she interviewed people who were doing things she thought were interesting. Over the years, I met a lot of these people and many of them wanted to "fix" me so they could take the credit for transforming me. They wanted to put me on a pedestal and say, "Look what I did! Isn't she awesome?" My attitude was, "How can you say anything about me? I'm shit. I'm nothing." At the same time, I knew I was something. We all are. But it pissed me off that they wanted to fix me so they could take credit for it. I resisted it all.

My mom and her friends wanted me to get interested in the things they were interested in.

> They would say, "Come on, Donnielle, you're a fringe dweller just like us, admit it!"
>
> I'd say, "No I'm not!"
>
> They'd say, "You're psychic, you're intuitive. You're just like us."

"No, I'm not!"

"Yeah, you are. Just accept it."

"No, screw you. I'm not going to do that." I kept thinking to myself, "It has to be easier than they're making it."

After years of working in TV, I left my job to go to Utah and help my mother take care of my elderly grandparents. After my grandparents died, it was time for me to go back to work and earn some money. Taking care of my grandparents had been difficult, and I had gained even more weight.

I knew I would have been welcomed back at my TV station. The president of my parent company, which owned several television stations throughout the United States told me, "If you ever change your mind, we'll find you a position. Just let me know." But that's not what I wanted to do.

Whenever I thought about going back to work in television, I'd get an extreme nauseous feeling. It was the heaviness of that whole TV production thing. The thought of going back to TV made me go, "ugh." I couldn't do it—but I didn't know what I wanted to do. I said to my mom, "I'm tired of being in limbo. I need to do something. I need to start earning money. My life has to change!"

Access Consciousness

About that time, my mom's friend, a network chiropractor who had been on her radio show, contacted my mom and said,"I'm working with some people from Access Consciousness. I think you should have them on the radio show."

My mom said, "Tell me some more about it," and she decided to interview them on her show.

One morning, my mom said to me, "The guests who are going to be on my show tomorrow are running our Bars[i] in exchange for being on the show."

I said, "What are Bars? What are you talking about?"

She said, "I'm not sure, but they'll talk to us about it before they do it."

My reaction was, "Now what crap have you gotten me into? I don't want to have my Bars run." But I went with my mom to find out what the Bars were in spite of my concern.

We went over to the house where mom's friend, Steve, was and he started talking with us about the Bars.

He said, "The brain is like a computer, and the Bars defrag your hard drive, get rid of unnecessary files, and give you a fresh, new slate." When Steve started comparing the Bars to a computer program, I sat up and went, "What?" I've always thought about computers and the brain in that way, and I have always loved computers. I had even thought to myself, "If I could write the correct program, I could shift myself."

The second the inspiration was there, I said, "Uh-oh, I've got to get out of here," but I was there, so I agreed to have my Bars run. It's a hands-on process that uses a light touch on the head of thirty-two contact points that correspond to different aspects of one's life.

The Bars are all about receiving, and I didn't receive very well. I had actively cut off receiving of any kind—receiving sexual energy from men, receiving compliments, receiving *me.* I didn't receive anything. I didn't receive money. I barely received air to breathe. So I was not comfortable during the Bars session, to say the least.

i See the Glossary.

> Steve said to my mom, "We'd like you to have Dr. Dain Heer from Access Consciousness on the show. He would call in, and you would interview him over the phone."
>
> Mom said, "Okay, that's cool." Steve started on mom's Bars, and while I was waiting, my mom asked if I would call Dain to set up the interview.
>
> I called, and he answered. I said, "Hello, could I speak to Dr. Heer?"
>
> He said, "This is Dain."
>
> I said, "This is Donnielle with the radio show," and we went through the particulars. I could feel his amusement—not that I was admitting I could sense anything over the phone. We finished and I said, "Okay, thank you for your time. I'll talk to you tomorrow."
>
> He paused and said, "It was very nice to meet you."
>
> I was taken aback. I said, "Yeah, you too. I'll talk to you tomorrow."

I hung up the phone. I was sitting outside on a bench in the sun, and I said, "Crap, I'm in so much trouble. I cannot hide from this man." That was my first thought. I actually said it out loud.

The next morning, Steve and Dain were on the radio show. Steve was in the studio, and Dain called in. I was behind the scenes, running the board and pushing the buttons, just the way I liked. Mom was interviewing Dain. I thought, "I can't wait for this interview to be done, because I've got to get away from this stuff." What I knew about Access Consciousness made sense to me, and my reaction was that I must run away. It terrified me at first because I knew I could change. I was at the crossroads of "Do I actually want to do this—or do I want to continue hiding? How much limbo do I want to stay in? Do

I want to stay here and whine about being in limbo—or do I want to change?" Plus, the thought that there was somebody who could see me was not fun for me.

After the radio interview, Steve said they were having a Bars class. I was not able to go to that class, but I blurted out, "I have to learn this stuff. I'd like to go to another class."

My mom said, "Huh?" She was shocked.

It shocked me too. It was as if my body said it. Who just said that? Crap. I had just put myself on their radar. I gave them my name and number.

After the interview, Dain gifted my mother with three sessions. At the time, we had no idea what a huge gift that was. We didn't know anything about Access Consciousness or Dain.

Mom had a phone session with Dain, and after the session, she said, "My daughter and I want to learn this. What do we need to do?"

He said, "Maybe I can get someone to come up from Las Vegas. There are a couple of facilitators there."

Then he said, "Do you know what? I have three days open next week. Why don't I come up and teach you guys?"

The next day, he said, "We're going to put a big class together while I'm there. We'll do a Foundation/Level One Access class, and I'll help to rewrite the course manual, because we update it all the time."

The date was two weeks out. I was thinking, "I'm not ready. Two weeks is too soon. No, he's going to see me, and I'm going to change. No!" Yet at the same time, I knew I'd be there.

The word got out that Dain was facilitating the class, and a lot of people came from California. About 25 of us showed up. When Dain came in on the morning of the class, I was sitting in my chair looking down. I didn't want to look at him. He picked my mother out of the crowd and gave her a hug. Then he came up the row I was sitting in to give me a hug. I finally looked up at him and went, "Shit! Oh no!" I couldn't look at his eyes. I knew he could see me. He started the class right off the bat. It was two weeks earlier that I had heard about Access Consciousness for the first time, and here I was in the Foundation Class. Dain started off with verbal processing[ii] and I was thinking, "What the hell have I gotten myself into?"

It turned out to be an interesting class. I didn't go because I wanted to lose weight. I didn't go because I wanted to change my body. That was the last thing on my mind. I went because I knew I needed change in my life. What I had learned about Access Consciousness was that it was fast and easy and great change was possible—if you chose it. It was the first method I had come across that empowered you. It's all about you. They give you the tools, but it's your choice to use them. If you don't use them, that's your choice, too. I thought, "Cool. This is all about me." I liked that.

During the class, Dain made mention of some people who had changed their bodies by using Access Consciousness tools. They let go of limitations, energetic bonds, barriers, and limitations that kept change from happening. I thought, "If someone else can do that, I can do it, too."

At the end of the third day of class, my older sister and her family were in town. My mom and I met them for dinner at our favorite Thai restaurant.

> After dinner, my sister asked Mom, "What kind of classes did you and Donnie go to?"

ii See the Glossary.

> My mom told her, and my sister said, "For the first time I can remember, Donnie didn't have that 'buzz' about food."

She had noticed—not that we had ever talked about it—that whenever I ate meals with others, I was always very cautious about what I ate and about how much food I took. I was very intense about eating, because I was intent on avoiding judgment. She could feel the energetic pulses of me wanting food and not wanting it—and she noticed that change in me—the absence of the "buzz"—even before I did.

We didn't talk specifically about food in the class. Becoming thinner has been a result of becoming more conscious and more aware in my life. I never set out to lose weight. I did say, "Oh! Being more in communion with my body, I could do that!" I began to ask questions about all the places I had limited myself. I started with my unhappiness, which was the most obvious thing. Then I asked, "What am I most unhappy about?" The answer was, "My body. I'm fat, and I feel ugly. I know I can be more." It wasn't that I wanted to change my body so I could be happy. I just wanted to stop hiding.

Getting Embodied

After the class, I bought the CD recording of the class so I could listen to it again. Most Foundation/Level One classes are not recorded because they are taught by facilitators like me, and the facilitators never think about doing it. But using the recordings was such a benefit for me that I now always record the classes I facilitate. I would listen to Dain's class and something would hit me, so I'd stop the CD, play it back again, and use the clearing statement on whatever came up. I would go down that path, wherever it took me, clearing whatever came up, and then I'd start listening to the class again.

Using the clearing statement is like opening up trenches in a pond filled with green, stagnant water. The energy is locked in, and it can't move. There is no outlet for it. The clearing statement opens a channel and moves the energy out. You're no longer stuck in that energy, that stagnation—you're in the flow and where there is constant change and fresh energy. It doesn't matter if the limitation was made five days ago or five million years ago. The clearing statement goes back and unlocks and reverses the energy that is held in place so you can reclaim who you were before you accepted that limitation. It's not living from the past; it's unlocking yourself from the past.

If a strange energy came up or I felt uncomfortable in my body for any reason, I would ask, "What is this? What's going on?" Sometimes I would have an awareness of what it was; other times I wouldn't know. I'd say, "Well, whatever that is, destroy and uncreate it." You don't have to know what something is to clear it. You don't have to define it. That's the beauty of Access.

One day after I had been doing some clearing, I had a conversation with my body for the first time since I was a kid. I apologized to it for ignoring it, abusing it, stuffing it full of food, starving it, and generally not listening to it. I told it I would change what I was doing, I would listen to it, and I would acknowledge it. I thanked it for continuing to try to talk to me even when I wasn't paying attention. I said I was grateful to it for not kicking me out or giving up on me.

During that conversation, I began to have a sense of *having* a body. I was alone in my office, and I let all my barriers down. I said out loud, "I have a body." Previously my body was just a thing I draped clothes on. It was a piece of meat I lugged around. I began to see it for the beauty it is and how much of this reality I had been missing because there was no communication. I promised to not judge it anymore.

Another night something big came up while I was making my bed. It was 10 p.m. I stopped, I sat down on the floor, and I did verbal processing until 3:30 in the morning. As you do the verbal processing, one layer gets uncovered, then another layer gets uncovered. Boom-boom-boom. I went to all the places I had tried to hide in my life and all the reasons I didn't want to be seen.

I went all the way back to being a brand new freshman in high school. During my freshman year, I had a huge fight with a girlfriend, and we never talked to each other again. As I sat there on the floor in my room, I used the clearing statement on the judgments, decisions, computations, and conclusions I had made at that time.

Twenty-four hours later—it had been 17 years since I was a freshman in high school—I got an email on Facebook from this same girlfriend, Nicole.

> She said, "Hey, is this Donnie from high school?"
>
> I didn't react with, "Ugh. Nicole." I said, "Wow, Nicole. How weird. Isn't that fun?" I replied, "Hey, how are you doing? Nice to talk to you. It's been so long."
>
> In her next email, she said, "I don't remember why we fell away from each other, but if I had anything to do with it, I truly apologize."

That was fascinating to me. I vividly remembered the fight and cleared it using the Access tools, and then twenty-four hours later, she found me on Facebook and apologized. I had shifted energetically, and it set us both free. I thought, "Holy crap! This shifting energy stuff is pretty amazing."

There is a greatness to embodiment. Embodiment is this entire reality, and our bodies are the key to fully experiencing it. If you're happy, where do you feel it? You feel it in your body. If you're frightened, even if you don't know why you're frightened, how do you feel it? You feel it in your body. You feel the sun, the wind, and the rain through your body. Think how much you would miss if you didn't have your body with you! I started opening up to that and being grateful for my body—even when it was very large. I started to look at all it gives me every day. The feeling of my clothes, the pleasure of petting a cat—all that is experienced through my body. I started being grateful, and I stopped judging it. I stopped thinking, "I have to be perfect." What's perfect anyway?

I made plans to go to an Access Consciousness Level Two and Three Classes in California and to Costa Rica for the seven-day Access Consciousness event, which was four months away. I told my body, "I promise to do more fun things with you. I'll go horseback riding when we're in Costa Rica," which was an option that was available. I could almost feel us riding as the wind was going by. I realized it was my body saying, "Yeah! Okay! Let's go do that!" I began to feel and hear my body's responses for the first time. It was so gentle, nurturing, and warm that I said, "I am so sorry that I spent my entire life ignoring you." It was like re-introducing myself to my body. It knew me, and I was letting myself say *hi* to it.

Asking Questions

As I went about my day, I asked a lot of questions, did the processes I learned in the Access classes, and used the POD/POC clearing statement on whatever came up. One question I used often was, **"Where am I creating limitations around my body? Where am I judging my body?"** I might respond with, "It's too fat." Then I'd say:

> *Okay, everything that is, everywhere I bought into that, all the decisions, judgments, conclusions, computations, projections, separations, expectations or rejections, past lifetimes, present, future, other dimensionalities, destroy and uncreate it. Right and wrong, good and bad, POD and POC, all nine, shorts, boys, and beyonds*[iii]*.*

iii This is the clearing statement. See the Glossary and Chapter 5 for more information.

Energy, Space, and Consciousness Processes

I also used the energy, space, consciousness (ESC) processes every day. They are great go-to processes simply because that's what *we* are. We are energy, space, and consciousness. I would ask, "What energy, space, and consciousness can I be, to be in total oneness and communion with my body?" Then I would use the POD/POC clearing statement:

> *Everything that doesn't allow that to show up times a godzillion, destroy and uncreate it all. Right and wrong, good and bad, POD and POC, all nine, shorts, boys, and beyonds.*

"What energy, space, and consciousness can my body and I be, to generate the body we desire and truly be?"

> *Everything that doesn't allow that to show up times a godzillion, destroy and uncreate it all. Right and wrong, good and bad, POD and POC, all nine, shorts, boys, and beyonds.*

"What energy, space, and consciousness can my body and I be that would allow us to be and appear exactly as we would like to be and appear?"

> *Everything that doesn't allow that to show up times a godzillion, destroy and uncreate it all. Right and wrong, good and bad, POD and POC, all nine, shorts, boys, and beyonds.*

Size 16 to Size 6

I was a very tight size 16 during the Foundation/Level One class I took with Dain. Four months later, when I went to California to take the Level Two and Three Class, I was wearing a size 8. Two days after this class, I went to the seven-day event in Costa Rica, and by end of the seven days, I was a size 6. I went from size a 16 to a size 6 in four months. This defied everything I had ever learned about bodies, health, and nutrition. I was taught that the only way to lose weight was two pounds a week. The conventional view was that if I had dropped that much weight that fast, I should have been flabby—which I wasn't. And I should not have been healthy—which I was.

People ask me, "How much weight did you lose?" I have no idea. I have not weighed myself in more than three years. I don't care what the scale says. It doesn't matter. Your weight can fluctuate pounds a day because of what you've eaten or the moisture in the air or whatever. Focusing on your weight is just a way to limit you, control you, and make you feel bad.

Peanut M&Ms

People also ask me if I changed the way I ate. I did, to a degree, but not from a deprivation point of view. Yes, my portions decreased, but not because I was counting calories or controlling my portions. I simply ask my body what it wants to eat and how much it wants—and that's what we have. So it's just, "Oh, you're done. Okay. Do you require anything else?" Maybe an hour later it will want something else. I let it do what it wants. Some days it wants to eat very little, some days it wants to eat a lot. Some days it wants to eat later. Some days it doesn't want to eat in the morning. It is interesting to see.

Some of what I did flies in the face of what I was taught about nutrition. For instance, I think peanut M&Ms are a complete food. I carry them with me in my computer bag. They contain sugar, salt, and protein. What more do you need in the world? People who are into nutrition say white sugar is bad for you, saturated fat is bad for you, and those peanuts are bad for you because they're rancid. According to the wisdom of this reality, peanut M&Ms are a horrible food, but when I eat them, my body sings. I stop when my body doesn't desire them any longer.

We spend our lives thinking, "There's a plate of food in front of me; I need to finish it." I don't do that anymore. A good way to know when your body is done eating a food is that the flavor changes. It's one of the ways your body communicates with you to tell you it has had enough.

I had never had a cup of coffee before I did Access Consciousness. I was raised Mormon, and if you're Mormon, you don't drink coffee! I remember being in the grocery store as a kid with my mom. We'd walk down the coffee aisle, and she would say, "I hate the coffee aisle." Even then I loved the smell, but it was wrong to like it. Mormon! You're not supposed to drink coffee. After I started doing Access Consciousness classes, I was visiting a friend in New York and I walked into a Starbucks with her. I said, "I think I'll have some coffee, too! Let's put some chocolate into it. Body, do you want some?" It said, "Yeah, yeah, yeah!" Now that I'm listening to my body, I love coffee. And curry. I used to hate curry with a fiery passion. Now I love it.

Access Consciousness Tools

I do muscle testing the way Gary and Dain teach it before I eat things. Say I have some nuts. I stand up with my ankles together, holding the nuts in a bowl in front of my solar plexus and I ask, "Body, do you want to ingest this?" or "Body, do you require this?" I have to loosen my knees a little or else I cheat. If the body leans forward, it's a *yes*. If it leans backward, it's a *no*. That's how it works for me. Everybody receives energy differently. When I facilitate body classes, I say, "I can tell you how I receive information, but it may be different for you. Your body might want to show you in a different way. You can ask the body, 'Body, show me what's a yes for you. Body, show me a *no*.'"

I also use the Access Heavy/Light tool. If something feels heavy, it's a lie or it's not right, don't do it. If it feels light, it's a truth for you. The more willing I became to receive information from my body, the easier it got. For me, *no* is a heaviness on my chest, and a *yes* is a lightness, which is a slight flush on my neck. It feels happy. I use the Heavy/Light tool, not just with food, but with finding what's true for me and for making changes in my life.

I ask questions such as, "Body, do you want to wear this today?" or "Body, what do you want for lunch?" Sometimes I get an image of what my body wants, like the leftover Thai food in the refrigerator, and I say, "Okay! That's what we'll have." Sometimes my body isn't hungry, and I respect that. I don't eat just because I'm supposed to. And I don't eat something because someone else tells me I should! If I don't feel light and happy after a meal, I know that, chances are, I didn't eat what my body wanted. It has nothing to do with quantity.

It's about being in a constant state of awareness. It's being willing to say, "Oh, that feels funny. What is it?" For instance, I'd find myself at the grocery store, starting to get that old, tense "buzzy" feeling about food again. Should I be eating this? Should I not be eating this? The grocery store would be full of people who were also doing their own freak outs about food, so I would stop, lighten up, and use tools such as *Who Does This Belong To?*[iv] and *Return It To Sender With Consciousness Attached.*[v] If something didn't lighten up for whatever reason, I knew there was probably a lie there, so I'd say, "Wherever I'm buying this as real and true, whatever this is, destroy and uncreate it."

iv See Chapter 4.

v See Chapter 9.

Body, What Do You Want to Look Like?

In one of the Access classes, we did an exercise called Body, What Do You Want to Look Like? I got an instant picture of Marilyn Monroe in her heyday, with the boobs, the waist, and the hips. I've always kind of known that's what my body wanted to look like. I remembered a time when I was very young. I was lying on my stomach on an ottoman, legs dangling, watching a show on TV about a sexy-looking woman who used her body to hurt people. I made a decision at that point that I never wanted to use my body to hurt anybody—and to me, that meant I couldn't have a sexy-looking body. I became unable to be my sexual self because I had equated harming people with being attractive and sexy! I was in Access Consciousness for about a year before I remembered that little tidbit. You don't always remember things right away. You have to get rid of some of the layers first. After I saw that, I felt so much more free, because that barrier wasn't there anymore. I had spent my life trying not to attract men and worrying about hurting people. Every time someone was attracted to me, I thought, "But no! What if I hurt you?" It's a crazy point of view, but it worked. I stopped attracting people.

Is This Really Possible?

As the weight came off, sometimes I'd think, "Is this really possible?" My clothes are loose, but I ate peanut M&Ms and Doritos yesterday, and I had a Coke.

According to this reality, I should not be losing weight. I'd ask, "Okay, Body, is it real that I'm losing weight?"

And it would say, "Yeah! It is."

Other times I was tempted to say, "This is fake. It's not real. It won't last." Then I'd say, "Wait a minute. Ask a question. Who does this belong to? What is this?

Can I change it? How do I change it?" I discovered that every time these fears came up, I was disconnected from my body.

Molecular De-Manifestation

A friend of my mother's thought I was losing weight too fast. She said, "You're releasing too many toxins into your body. You need to do a gall bladder cleanse.

You need to do this. You need to do that."

I said, "Actually, I feel better than I used to!"

In the Level Three Class, I learned about a process called Molecular De-Manifestation[vi] and the things you could do with it. I thought, "I wonder what else is possible with that process." Every night before I went to bed, I did Molecular De-Manifestation of the fat and the toxic chemicals in my body. I had no idea whether it would do anything. My attitude was, "What the hell. If it works, cool. If it doesn't work, cool." I wanted to see what would happen. I was just playing and experimenting with my body.

My clothes had gotten so big for me that I had to go shopping for new ones. It was a joy to discover the things I could wear. One day when I was shopping for something to wear to a friend's wedding, I saw a halter dress made of flowing fabric with white and purple flowers on it. The hem was higher in the front than the back. It had a great look to it. When I saw it, my body went "Whoosh!" and I said, "No! It's sleeveless, and it's a halter. I can't wear that! I can't show my bare arms!" I had to do some POD and POCing before I could even put the dress on. I took two different sizes of the dress into the dressing room, and when I put on the larger size, I thought it was kind of cute. I was shopping with my mom at the time and she said, "I think you should try the smaller one." I slipped on the smaller one, tied it around my

vi See the Glossary for more information about Molecular De-Manifestation.

neck, and my body started to sing. I went, "Ahh!" and all the angst went away because I could feel my body saying, "Yeah! This is what I want to wear!" It's a great dress, and I have a great wrap to go with it. That's probably the first time I went from tomboyish—hair pulled back in a pony tail, no make-up, loose fitting jeans, and T-shirts that I wore until they were threadbare—to showing off and playing with the way I dressed. Now I love adorning my body and wearing beautiful clothes and jewelry. I still don't have the "perfect" size 2 or size 4 body, whatever that is, but I'm enjoying my body. Isn't that the whole point?

I now touch my body more, not necessarily in a sexual way—I just touch it and caress it. I get more frequent massages. There's no more embarrassment about taking my clothes off. I don't care. Look at me. And I enjoy the movement of my body. I ask it, "Body, how do you want to move?" It enjoys the stretching of yoga and pilates. When I do those things now, I'm with my body, and I enjoy the movement down to my fingertips instead of because I think I need to tighten up or that it will make me look better. I do it when my body wants to do it.

Just Use the Tools

People have asked if it took me a long time to develop this way of being with my body. In the grand scheme of things, the answer is no. I spent 34 years ignoring my body. Change can come quickly if you allow it. It didn't require discipline. That's the joyous thing about Access Consciousness and listening to your body. There is no discipline. There's no regimen. You just have to use the tools.

In the diet world, you have to do this, this, and this. In the metaphysical world you have to use this prop or this herb or that ritual. With Access Consciousness, there's none of that. It's, "Which tool do I need to use now?" There was no exercise, no special way of eating, no deprivation, no rigorous training. Whatever my body wanted, I did it. It was just the simple ease of listening to my body. Do you want to eat? No. Okay. Are you hungry? No. Okay. Are you thirsty? Yes. Okay.

Ease

There's such a sense of ease about life now. It's not a burden to listen to my body. It took much more energy and effort to work against it. I have become more aware of everything with the assistance of my body. I feel energy through my body now. Some people only listen to their body when they feel pain. There's another way. Your body is communicating all the time. Pain is the last straw. It's like the body is saying, "I'm going to turn up the intensity until you hear me." And the intensity eventually turns into pain. What if you could listen to your body before that? That's what I did—and it creates ease. It's fun, light, and joyful.

One of the big changes that occurred has been my willingness to be seen. In the past, as I've said, I was in hiding. I had spent so much of my life off camera and off the microphone. I would run the sound board for the various radio shows at the station where I now have a show, but I wouldn't speak. Once I was playing a pre-taped show, and all I had to do was go on and say, "You are about to listen to a pre-recorded show. If you want to get in touch with ___, you can contact him at ____," and then hit *play*. Ten seconds worth of copy. I was nervous for a week about doing this. I had to write it down, and when I said it on the air, my voice trembled, and I was sweating like a pig. Now you can't get me to shut up! I do a radio show every Saturday, and I facilitate Access Consciousness classes.

> Recently my mom called me at 10:30 on a Friday night and said, "I'm sick. I can't do the interviews on my shows tomorrow morning. Will you host them?"
>
> I said, "Sure, no problem."
>
> She said, "Dr. So-and-so is on at 10."
>
> I said, "Okay, what are we talking about?"
>
> "Hypothyroidism."
>
> I don't know anything about hypothyroidism. I thought, "Okay. I can ask questions."
>
> She said, "At 11, an herbalist is going to be on the phone and we were going to talk about radiation."
>
> I thought, "Okay, I know nothing about these topics, but I will go on and talk about them for two hours, no problem."

I could do this, because I like being me now. I'm happy. I don't mind being seen, looked at, or even judged. Judge me and have a good time! I can choose not to have it affect me. Since I'm more comfortable being me, I can talk, people can see me, and I walk through the world differently. I get attention, which used to terrify me. It used to be, "Don't look at me!" Now it's okay. I don't mind being seen. I'm willing to receive all of that. I'm willing to be heard. I'm willing to be the gift to the world that I can be, because we're all a gift to the world.

There's such a sense of ease about life now.
It's not a burden to listen to my body.
It took much more energy and effort to work against it.

Part Two

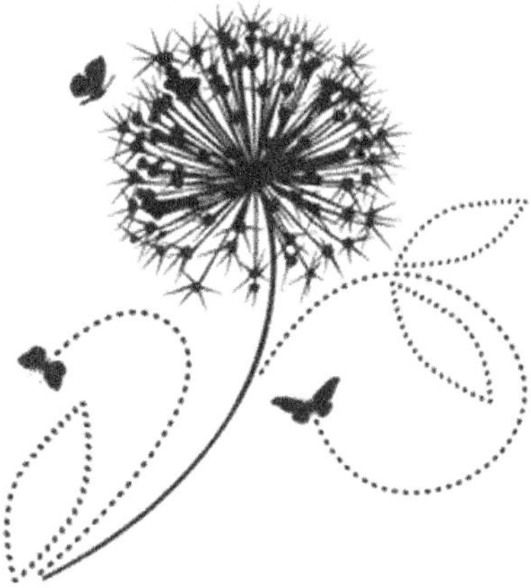

by Gary M. Douglas

Chapter 2

Embodiment

Your body will take care of you if you listen to it.
Your body actually wants to take care of you!

You, as an infinite being, are energy, space, and consciousness. You are actually the space between the molecules of your body. You keep trying to create yourself as solid and real—but that's not what you are. What if you were willing to be the energy, space, and consciousness you truly are? What if you were willing to be nothing but the space between the molecules? What if you had the capacity, the power, and the potency to hold those molecules together? The truth is you do.

Your Body

Someone recently asked me, "What is the relationship between a body and a being? I know that I am with this body—but do I own this body or is this body just a part of me?"

I asked her to do this exercise, which I invite you to try as well:

> *Close your eyes. Reach out and touch the outside edges of you. Not the outside edges of your body, but the outside edges of you, the infinite being. Reach out energetically and touch the edges of you. Go out to the farthest reaches of where you, as a being, are. Now go farther. Are you there too? Could a being that big fit inside a human-sized body? No. Your body is inside you, the being. It's not the other way around; you are not part of your body. You are the creator of your body. You create it every moment of every day with every point of view you take.*

You Embody Everything Here

Your body is not just a thing by itself. It's not that there's you and your body and then there's the rest of the world. It's that you embody everything here. Your body is not somehow separate from the rest of your life. You try to take your body along for the ride rather than realizing that you and your body are a creation and an embodiment of this reality.

Just about every religion on the planet has the point of view that your body is a pile of meat that you're supposed to use, and your soul is what is valuable. We are repeatedly told by churches, cults, and religions that the soul is superior to the body—the soul is the only thing that's valuable. This way of thinking creates a separation between you and your body. Your body is not less than you. Your body is part of you. It has amazing capacities. It can do remarkable things. What if you included the magic of your body—and the magic of everything—in your life? Your body has to be incorporated into the oneness of you, as part of you, because it is part of who and what you are.

You have to be in gratitude for your body. You can function from a whole different place when you are grateful for your body. Are you grateful for your body? Or do you treat it disrespectfully? Do you communicate with your body about what it wants? Or do you say, "I want to go here, I want to go there, I want to eat this, I want to drink that, I want to sleep with that person"? When you do this, you are being inconsiderate of your body. You are defying your body and fighting with it instead of *being* with it. And when you're in defiance and resistance of your body, you can't be in gratitude for it—nor can you communicate with it.

If you treated your lover like that, would your lover stick around or would he or she bug off? Your lover would bug off! What if you worked *with* your body? What does working with your body look like? Well, for starters, you are grateful for it. You communicate with it. You ask it questions to find out what it needs and desires—and you listen for the awareness that will come to you as its response.

When you begin to listen to your body, something entirely different can show up for you.

If you haven't been listening to your body, now is the time to begin. Start by asking questions and then listen intently. Let your body show you what it needs. You may not realize it, but your body, like any other animal, knows exactly what it requires. It knows when it wishes to eat and what it wishes to eat. Its awareness of what it needs is far greater than yours.

I had a wonderful horse that I used to take on trail rides in the Santa Barbara foothills. At one point, I noticed that whenever we were out on the trail, he continuously ate dandelions, but I didn't pay much attention to it. Then once when I was out of town, he came down with colic, which is an intestinal disorder, and he was taken to the vet. The vet discovered he had a fatty tumor that took up 18 feet of his intestines. They removed the tumor and he survived. I later found out that dandelions have many different medicinal uses. They help with the digestive process, contribute to eliminating fatty tissue in the body, and supposedly help with cancer. My horse had been eating those dandelions to keep the tumor from becoming a problem.

Dogs, cats, horses, and all the critters on the planet eat whatever their body tells them to eat. When you see dogs or cats, which are basically carnivores, chewing on grass, you know they've got something going on in their body that needs solving. Your body has the same ability and awareness as a horse's, a dog's, or cat's. It knows what it needs and it will tell you—if you ask—and if you listen.

How Do You Treat Your Body?

If you're like most people, you choose to do things with your body that aren't nice to it. You may actually be very good at making your body suffer. Maybe you used to go out and get drunk, then go home with people you didn't like and who didn't like you. You would wake up the next morning and ask, "Why did I choose this?" Maybe you have woken up with way too many hangovers. Or maybe you tried to take drugs, sex, and rock 'n' roll to a new level so you could become enlightened. Or maybe it was something else. Unfortunately none of those things worked.

Do you work too hard? You know you're doing it—but you continue anyway. You say, "It's okay, I just have a little more to do. I won't quit, I'll keep going, going, going." Then not much later, you say, "Oh no, I now feel like crap." No, *you* don't feel like crap. Your *body* feels like crap. It wanted you to stop long ago, but you wouldn't listen. Many of the routine, normal things you do are immensely cruel to your body. You make things much tougher on your body than they have to be. You force your body to do things it doesn't want to do because you've decided it's supposed to do them. All of those things are being mean to your body.

Your dog would run away from home if you treated it the way you treat your body. If your body were a dog, it would leave you and find somebody else who would take better care of it. And dogs don't leave people easily; they take lots of abuse. You should pamper your little body the way you pamper your dog. Scratch it behind the ears, rub its chest and belly, and tell it what a good body it is. You need to get up in the morning and say, "Thanks, body, for putting up with me. I love you."

A friend of mine had a female Tantric teacher come to see him. She wanted to have sex with him, but he couldn't get it up. He was horrified. He did everything under the sun that usually did to get it up, but it wasn't happening. He asked me what was going on.

> I asked him, "Do you remember what she said the last time she was here?"
>
> He said, "No. What did she say?"
>
> I said, "She said she was ready to be a single mom. Is she coming to get impregnated?"
>
> He said, "Oh, my God! Yes!" He paused for a moment then started to lovingly stroke his chest and say, "Good body, good body, good body!"
>
> Now when he can't get it up, he asks, "Is this person going to get pregnant?" Every time he asks he gets a *yes.* The body knows, "This is going to result in a pregnancy."

Do You Work Against Your Body?

Who do you know that is kind to their body? Watch people who work out. They work the crap out of their body until it's almost "perfect," and then they judge it and tell it that it is a pile of debris. They are training themselves not to be kind and not to see what is true for their body. Have you trained yourself to not be kind to your body and to not see your body as it would like to be?

There are hundreds of ways we work against our body. Watch people walking down the street, including people that are supposedly into their bodies, like jocks and weightlifters, whether they are guys or girls. Watch skinny people, anorexic-looking people and heavy-set people, not to mention people the size of refrigerators. Do they seem to enjoy their bodies and appreciate them? Are they aware of how their bodies move? No. Most people work *against* their bodies rather than *for* them. Most people abuse their bodies horribly.

When I met my first wife, who was a dancer, she ate nothing but tuna fish and pickles because she was trying to get skinny. She would work like crazy, belly dancing, tap dancing, and doing whatever she did. It was never about the joy of her body—ever. It still isn't. Now she's got nothing but pain and disability in her body. That's where you end up if you go down that road. It doesn't have to be that way.

I know a woman who was involved in a cult where there was a great deal of stress, duress, and pressure to get work done. She often went without sleep for one, two, or three nights in a row in order to complete the projects she was working on. Sometimes when her exhaustion became overwhelming, she would lie down on the floor under her desk to take a short nap. Then she'd get up and start working again.

That's what I call being a terrorist to your body. Many of us have done things like this to our body at one time or another. Have you trained yourself to be a terrorist to your body? Any time you take a fixed point of view about anything that has to do with your body, you've already planned the unkindness you're going to deliver. All the ways you've decided you have to live, all the ways you've decided things are going to be, and all the things you've decided are going to happen are the ways you plan to do what is unkind to your body. You leave it out of the equation by never asking it what it wants. You don't listen to it or act out of consideration for it.

Being Kind to Your Body

You may think being kind to your body is resting or eating sugar or some such thing, but being kind is more than that. Being kind to your body is knowing when to stop and when to listen. It's knowing that if you truly listen to what's going on in your life you won't have repeating disasters to deal with. Every time you drink something your body doesn't want, every time you eat something when your body isn't hungry, every time you choose to go against what your body is saying, how mean are you being to your body? You are being as mean as a snake with a knot in its tail.

What If You Added 10 Percent More Kindness to Your Body?

One of the ways I am kind to my body is to be very aware. This contributes to my body in many different ways. For example, when I'm very aware as I go through my day, I accomplish a great deal. This is being kind to my body because it means I have more time to rest and play and to create and generate a sense of ease and joy in my life. Instead of overworking my body, instead of hurting my body, I create ease and peace in my body with everything I do and everything that occurs. This helps me get everything done more quickly than I would by forcing myself to do things.

Recently I woke up one morning and I knew I had to have some work done on my car. Every time I started it up, the "change oil" light came on and then instantly went off. I could easily have ignored it for another week or two until the car refused to start, but I decided to be aware and take it in to the mechanic. I wanted to have it fixed before it broke down, and I had the auto club coming out to rescue me.

While I waited for my assistant to pick me up at the mechanic's, I decided to walk down the street to an antique shop I liked. Before I got to the shop, I saw a carpet store I hadn't previously noticed. One of the things I wanted to accomplish that morning was to find a store that carried a certain kind of carpet. I had told a friend this carpet would be perfect in her house, but, unfortunately, she couldn't find it anywhere. So, I went into the carpet store and found the exact carpet I had told my friend about without having to drive all over town. Boom! I had the awareness that allowed me to find the carpet in the moment the store presented itself. Most of us don't pay attention to the awareness that our body, our car, and our whole life are trying to give us—but from my point of view, it's always a kindness to our body when we do.

Here's a question you can ask yourself every morning, **"What 10 percent of kindness can I be to my body today?"** There are a thousand different ways you can be 10 percent more kind to your body. We talked about being kind to your body in a recent Access Consciousness class, and a woman said, "When I asked what 10 percent of kindness I could be to my body, it said it would like more warmth. I realized I've been ignoring it when it's cold. It's an unkind habit I've gotten into."

Most of us have gotten into a habit of ignoring our bodies. We say to ourselves, "I'm cold, but I can stand it." Is that kind? No! Is it being aware of your body? No! Is it asking your body a question? No! It's making a decision that excludes your body. Your body knows when it needs to be warmer.

Before I left for a trip to Montreal last spring, I found out what the temperature was going to be. The prediction was 38 to 50 degrees. That's cold by my body's standards, so I took an overcoat, a jacket, a sweater, my scarf and, my gloves. That's being kind.

There's also the warmth of being touched that your body desires. If your body desires to be touched more, it means you have to be willing to touch more! Most of us think that we want somebody to touch us. Sometimes you have to touch others for them to be willing to touch you, and you have to be willing to touch yourself. How often do you refuse to touch others while desiring to be touched yourself?

Enjoying Your Body

You created your body; so why aren't you enjoying it? What if the purpose in life was to enjoy your body every moment of every day? Are you doing that? If you wake up in the morning, it's time to live! Get busy and enjoy yourself! Don't do things you don't wish to do! Do all the things you'd like to do. Ask:

- *Body, what would you like to do today?*
- *Body, what would make you happy?*
- *Body, what would be fun for you to do today?*

Most people never ask these questions. They say things like, "Oh, I want to dance." But they never ask their body if it wants to dance. Or they say, "I want to lie in the sun forever," but they don't ask their body if that's what it would like!

It's amazing what can happen when you are kind to your body and in communion with it. Communion is a sense of oneness with your body. You and your body work together within the structure of the whole world. There is no sense of separation between you, your body, and the rest of the world. You are connected to all things. It's the way you feel when you go out in the deep woods. You experience a sense of being part of everything there. You are not separate from anything. The woods nurture you—and you contribute to the woods. When you start to be in communion with your body at all times, there's a sense of peace that you get no other way.

The Joy of Embodiment

There's a reason to be here on this planet that relates to the joy of embodiment. It's a place we need to function from. You should have a level of communion with your body that allows you to enjoy it—but that doesn't seem to happen in this reality. This explains why we can't do magical things with our bodies. If we could see that there's a greatness in embodiment, we would have a totally different possibility in what we could create and generate.

What would happen if you were actually nice to you and nice to your body?

Chapter 3

Being Ambiguous

I invite you to be in communion with your body. Being ambiguous—asking questions—is the way to do that.

Ambiguous means unclear, uncertain, or vague. When you're being ambiguous, it means you haven't latched on to an answer or a conclusion. You haven't defined things. You haven't made decisions or judgments. You haven't decided what can—and cannot—be done. You're alert and aware. You are in the question—and when you are in the question, you are open to everything that is possible.

Many people have misidentified and misapplied that ambivalence and ambiguity are the same. They are not. ***Ambivalence*** is where you see the difference between two things. and you can't choose one or the other. It's being two-sided. You're limited. It's either this—or it's that. Those are the only options. ***Ambiguity*** takes you out of the either/or universe—and into possibility.

If you give up the ambiguity and possibility of being an infinite being, you lose some of your power and end up feeling like a finite being, subject to the whims and furies of outrageous fortune. But if you apply ambiguity to everything you do, you have infinite choices—because you aren't making anything finite.

For example, if you perceive a feeling or sensation, instead of calling it whatever you *think* it is, "Oh, my back aches" or "I feel tired," remain in ambiguity. Don't give it a name. Just ask, **"What can I do with this?"** This is a way to shift your perspective so you stop imposing judgments and decisions on your body. You say you are "feeling bad" or you "have a headache" or you "feel (whatever you decide to call the feeling)." When you define something in this way, you destroy the possibility of discovering what it truly might be. What if it's a non-cognitive awareness that you are having? Have you ever had moments where you get a feeling about something or you sense that something is not quite right, but you don't know what it is? That's a non-cognitive awareness. You start looking around, and you question more about what's happening—and then all of a sudden, you find out. That's functioning from non-cognitive awareness.

A few years ago, I was in Texas, driving with a friend in her car. I got a sense that we should stop for coffee, but I thought, "I don't need any coffee," and I kept driving. Right after that I got a sense that we should stop at an antique store

I saw—but it was closed. Then I came to a stoplight. There was a giant truck next to us. The light turned green, but the truck didn't move. I asked, "What's going on?"

I started to creep forward very slowly—and that's not the way I usually drive. I usually stomp on it. I am not a person who creeps forward slowly out in front of cars. As I was slowly moving forward, a car came out of nowhere, smashed into the front of my friend's car and kept going. It was a hit-and-run. I crept out because I *sensed* that something wasn't quite right—but I didn't know what it was. We weren't hurt—but we could have been if I had gone forward at a higher speed.

We all have moments of non-cognitive awareness like this. It wasn't that I could see something ahead of me; I didn't know why I was moving so slowly. There was no "reason" I crept forward so slowly—I just somehow knew I needed to be careful. When you function from non-cognitive awareness, everything becomes so much easier. We need to do this at all times. It's an important part of being ambiguous.

You've been taught your entire life that you're not supposed to have ambiguity. Ambiguity is considered wrong in this reality. You're supposed to have a fixed point of view. You're supposed to nail things down and define them. You are taught to believe that if you have a sufficient number of fixed points of view, then you really have something. I'm not sure what it is you're supposed to have with all those fixed points of view—but you're supposed to have *something.*

It's in your best interest to be ambiguous because when you're being ambiguous, you're living in the question. What if ambiguity is your primary way out of this reality? Do you know what? It is! It's the place from which you ask questions—which gives you greater awareness—which then creates greater possibility.

Say you have ten pounds more than you desire on your body. You might go into "Oh, this is terrible!" What kind of question is that? It isn't a question! It's a judgment. You tell your body, "You're wrong, bad, and terrible!" instead of asking it how you can change what's going on, which is being in the question. What do you do when somebody tells you you're wrong, bad, and terrible? Do you fight and resist and say, "F--- you, I will not change that!" Do you align and agree with them and say, "You're right, I am wrong, bad, and terrible." Or do you walk away? Are you walking away from your body—or fighting your body—or agreeing that it's in bad shape—rather than asking it a question? You need to go into an ambiguous place where you ask, "Okay, Body, what are we doing and how can we change this?"

Listen for the Awareness

When you ask your body a question, listen for the awareness—not the answer. An answer feels like a solidity; it's based on everyone else's point of view. An awareness is an expansive universe that creates more ease for you and your body. Sometimes it may take a couple of days or even a week or a month for the awareness to show up. Keep listening. Most people don't bother to ask a question of their body—but some do. They ask a question, but if the awareness doesn't come instantaneously they stop listening. You've got to be willing to listen. You might ask, "But why haven't I received an awareness yet?" or "When is the awareness coming?" or "How soon is it going to get here?" A better question would be, **"What would it take for me to have the awareness?"**

No Choice Universe

Someone recently said to me, "My mother's body is deteriorating. She just had an eye operation, which instead of improving her vision, left her blind in one eye. This means she can't drive, and I'm going to have to do a lot of additional things to help her. This is going to be very difficult for me, and I'm dreading it. What can I do to change the way I feel?"

I asked, "What about this have you decided is your responsibility?"

She replied, "I have decided it's my responsibility to help her and care for her."

I asked, "Is it actually your responsibility?"

She said, "I would like to be able to say no, but I keep saying yes because there is no one else to do it."

I asked, "Well, could you hire a driver for her?"

She said, "Oh, I see! I'm not looking at choices here."

This is an example of the problem you create when you don't ask questions. You decide you have to take responsibility for people. You jump directly to taking responsibility and you leave yourself no choice. But there is always a choice. You can replace the words *my mother* for any situation where you feel you have no choice; that is, anywhere you are in a no-choice universe. Your particular no-choice universe might have to do with your job or your money or your relationship. Or maybe it has to do with your body!

For the longest time, I could not understand why people would not ask questions. I couldn't understand why they would try to find the "right" answer, as if there were such a thing. Then I realized that people are unwilling to be ambiguous. As long as you're unwilling to be ambiguous, you aren't able to ask questions.

What Do You Think You Like?

A great deal of what we think we like has more to do with other people's reality than our own, because we're not willing to be ambiguous. We try to define ourselves based on what we like to eat, what we like to drink, what we like to do, or what we think is good. None of that has anything to do with reality. If you have absolutely no fixed point of view, you have total choice. But as long as you have an ounce of a fixed point of view, you have no choice.

It is a lot more fun to create your life like the characters in the movie *Fifty First Dates*, which is about a woman who has a condition where she can't remember anything about the previous day. She starts each day brand new with no judgments carried forward, so for her, every day is full of possibilities and adventure. She's not tied down by the decisions she made the day before. I recommend that you watch the movie 50 times to find out what it would be like to be on a first date with yourself and your body.

Being in Communion with Your Body

I'm inviting you to be in communion with your body. Being ambiguous—asking questions—is the way to do that. Be ambiguous about your body and with your body. Use questions like these:

- *What is this?*
- *What can I do with it?*
- *Can I change it and how do I change it?*
- *How do my body and I change it? You ask this question because you and your body are a connected item.*

Tool: Heavy or Light not Wrong or Right

When you are asking questions, look for whatever causes you to feel lighter. You're not looking for what's right or wrong. If yes feels lighter, that's your awareness of the energy of possibility. The first thought that goes through your head that feels light is your knowing. The second thought is the doubt you create in order to invalidate the fact that you do know. That thought will feel heavy.

Whatever is true is light and whatever is a lie is heavy. Stop when you hit a lie. Most people don't do this. They find something that's a lie and then they try to figure out what part of it is right or what part of it they chose. They then ask why they chose it—as though finding out why they chose it will get them out of it. We've been taught that there has to be a root cause and a reason for something. This is not the case. This is a lie.

You have to use this tool from the place of ambiguity. Don't decide what the answer is ahead of time. There are people who say, "That didn't make me feel light" so they can justify the reason they chose what they chose. Or they say,

"That feels heavy" as a reason not to choose what they've already decided not to choose. Don't decide in advance! Don't come to conclusions. Be in the question. Be ambiguous.

It's very simple. All you have to do is look at something and ask:

- *Is this making me feel light?*
- *If it isn't making you feel light, then it's not true. It's a lie.*
- *If it's a lie, let it go.*
- *Go back to what makes you feel light.*

Every question you ask creates the possibility and the life and living of your body.

Chapter 4

Judging Your Body

Whenever you take a fixed point of view,
all you will see is what matches your fixed point
of view.

Do you get up in the morning, look at yourself in the bathroom mirror, and say, "I look terrible this morning. "Who is that old man (or old woman) looking out of my eyes?" Or do you say, "This is too saggy. This is too draggy. This is not big enough, and that's too short"? These are judgments. What does judgment create? Judgment creates more judgment.

If you're like everyone else I've ever met, you have a love affair with judging yourself and your body. Your judgments are the way you create your body and the way you destroy your body. How do I judge me? Let me count the ways.

What you and most other people are doing right now is this: "My body doesn't look like (fill in the blank)." In the blank are all the things you use to judge your body. "My body doesn't look the way it did when it was 21. My body does not look like a sex machine. My body does not look like (you name it!)." These are the love potions you deliver to your body.

People judge their bodies mercilessly. They say, "I'm fat—or I'm skinny—and no one will ever be interested in me" or "If you're big, nobody wants you." These things are not true. There are a number of cultures where you're considered the hottest thing in the world if you've got a big, fat body. There are others cultures where if you're a Skinny Minnie, you're the greatest thing in the world. There are cultures (in this case, the culture is called "men") in which if you've got some serious cleavage, they don't care about the rest. There are also a lot of people who don't have judgments of bodies. They just enjoy whatever body is in front of them. They know that what's enjoyable is a body that's sensitive and willing to receive. What if you just loved your body? If you don't love your body, you can't have fun with it. You have to start by loving it. Do you ever look at your body and say, "Body, you're really nice. How do you put up with me?"

What do you want to create as your life? Do you want to have fun or do you want to judge your body? A woman who weighed 200 pounds came to an Access Consciousness class.

> She said, "I know you're saying I'm so fat that nobody will ever look at me."
>
> I said, "You have some weight on you, but you have created some seriously beautiful breasts. If you use that as a little leverage, take advantage of the assets you've created and show a little cleavage, you'll be surprised at what happens."
>
> She said, "I could never do that."

I asked, "Why not?"

She said, "Because that would make me a slut!"

I asked, "And why wouldn't you want to be a slut?"

She said, "Oh, it was my mother's point of view that it's bad to be a slut."

I said, "What if you didn't judge and you just used your cleavage to your advantage? You know, sluts have fun. Sluts do what they want. Sluts don't judge. They just enjoy themselves."

She called me a month later and said, "I have had more sex in the last month than I have had in the last ten years. I love you! I started wearing clothes that showed my cleavage and since then, I've had men chase me down on the freeway to get my telephone number and beg me to let them take me to dinner and have a good time with me. I am having more fun than I have had in my entire life! Thank you so much. I am a great, chesty slut."

Own the Greatness of Your Body

Have you bought the idea that a body is a wrong thing? Do you believe that the being is great, your body is wrong, and your soul is the only thing of value? That's the result of too many churches, cults, and religions! You are lying to yourself when you buy the wrongness of your body and refuse to be aware of what is truly possible. A radically different physical embodiment is the recognition that there is a greatness in embodiment. There is something about having a body that is of tremendous value. It's not a wrongness. You've got to be willing to own the frigging greatness of your body! When you go into the wrongness of your body, you don't acknowledge the potency you are, to have created it.

Your Point of View Creates Your Reality

There's a set of four novels by Lawrence Durrell called *The Alexandria Quartet.* Each novel presents a different person's point of view about a single set of events that took place before and during World War II. As you read, you begin to realize how different each person's point of view is from everybody else's. You also begin to see that it's only your point of view that creates your reality. It's not reality that creates your point of view.

> Recently I was talking with a woman who said, "I am judging my body less, and it's great. My body and I are having more fun. I don't see that it has changed much, but I keep getting unsolicited feedback from people who see my body very differently than I do."
>
> I said, "That's because they see you from their own point of view. Nobody sees the same thing. You can't see what is. You can only see what you judge it to be."

We create the structure, the form, and the significance of our bodies based on our judgments, as though judgment is a source of creation. The difficulty is that judgment is never a source of creation. It's simply a source of answers and more judgment.

The Mirror Is a Reflection of Your Judgment

I had a conversation with a friend about the novel, *The Portrait of Dorian Gray* by Oscar Wilde. In the story, an artist paints a portrait of a young man named Dorian Gray. One day as Dorian contemplates his portrait, he says:

> *How sad it is! I shall grow old, and horrible, and dreadful. But this picture will remain always young. It will never be older than this particular day of June.... If it were only the other way! If only it were I who was to be always young, and the picture that was to grow old!*

> *For that—for that—I would give everything! Yes, there is nothing in the whole world I would not give! I would give my soul for that!*

You can guess what happens. Dorian gives his soul to remain eternally youthful and beautiful. He then begins to commit ugly and destructive acts against others—and the face in the painting (which is hidden away in the attic) becomes terrifyingly old and ugly.

> I said to my friend, "You have to understand that you keep a portrait of yourself in the attic of your mind. It's called the mirror in your bathroom. This is where you create the ideas that you're uglier, older, fatter, or skinnier than you really are. You look at that portrait every day and compare your body to it—but the portrait only shows you a reflection of your judgments. That's all it can do. The mirror is nothing but a reflection of your judgments."

I have worked with a number of people who are anorexic, and I've noticed that when they stand in front of a mirror, all they see are their judgments of how fat they think they are. Overweight people who look in the mirror view their bodies through a kaleidoscope. All they see is one small area that is magnified and distorted. We all use the judgments of our bodies to create our bodies. Your body is designed and structured to follow your judgments. If you didn't have any judgment of your body at all, you wouldn't even notice what it looked like—ever! But we notice things and we judge them, and then we judge the things that we judge. What does this do? It creates our body. You use your potency and power to create (with your judgments) the structure of your body the way it is, instead of the way it could be or the way it would like to be.

Do you get up in the morning and ask, "How beautiful can you be today, my darling body?" Do you look in the mirror and ask, "Okay, Beauty, let's see what we can be"? No, you say, "Beauty, you're a beast." If your hair is getting thin, do you ask your body, "What do we need to do in order to grow more hair?" Do you listen for the awareness—or do you come to a conclusion, torture yourself and your body, and say, "Oh my God! We're losing our hair!" Everything you do with that creates greater hair loss, because that's where you're putting your energy. You make losing your hair real.

A while ago, I got up in arms because my hair was getting white. I thought it was ridiculous for me to have white hair. I thought I should be able to naturally turn it dark again. I got a bunch of homeopathic remedies for turning my hair dark and I took them, and then one day, I realized I had the point of view that it was wrong to have white hair. With my judgment, I was keeping the wrongness of my white hair in place. Somehow I had thought that using homeopathic remedies took away the wrongness of it, but they didn't change the energy of what I was creating. When I saw this, I said, "Who cares?" I'm now at peace with the color of my hair.

Allowance

You have to be in allowance of your body. Allowance is: Everything is just an interesting point of view. You don't resist or react to any judgment or point of view. You don't align or agree with any judgment or point of view. Everything is neither right nor wrong nor good nor bad. If nothing was right and nothing was wrong, what would you and your body be? You'd be whatever you chose to be. And you'd be happy!

Are you in loving allowance of your body? Or are you saying, "Well, yes, I'm in loving allowance of my body, except when it's fat in the wrong place and skinny in the wrong place and too short in the wrong place or too long in the wrong place"? That's not loving allowance. That's judgment!

Tool: Interesting Point of View

The antidote to judgment is "Interesting Point of View." Every time you encounter a judgment, no matter where it comes from, just say: **Interesting point of view or Interesting point of view that I have this point of view.**

What if you had no judgments of you? What if you had no thoughts, feelings, or emotions? You'd be totally mindless and totally aware. Now, some people think the mind is a good thing, but I beg to differ. Your mind can only do one thing—it defines what you already know. That's all it can do. It can't go beyond the limitations of this reality, which is another way of saying that it can't go beyond what everyone else thinks is true. What if you could have something different? What if you could do something different? What if you could be something different? You, as an infinite being, can go beyond the scope of everybody else's reality—if you choose it.

Other People's Judgments

You can buy other people's points of view, lock them into your body, and make yourself miserable if you wish. This is something we all do—and we're good at it. We receive someone else's thoughts—and then we bat them around as if they were our own. And to make things even crazier, we don't even pick up their thoughts accurately. It's as if we're playing that children's game called Telephone or Chinese Whispers. One person whispers into another person's ear and the second person hears something totally different from what the first person said. Person one says, "I'm such a bore." Person two hears, "I have to go to the store," and whispers it to person three, who hears, "I'm a whore," and so on. That's how it works. You apply the things you think you hear to your life and you use them to judge yourself. Do you see what a mess this gets you into? If you truly understand that 99,000 percent of the thoughts, feelings, and emotions that go through your head don't belong to you, you may stop taking on other people's points of view and judgments.

If you buy other people's points of view, you end up buying into the idea that this body is of no value or it doesn't look right or it is whatever they say it is! None of that is real; it's just your entrainment. Entrainment is something we do all the time. If women live together in the same house, they will eventually all be on the same monthly cycle. If you put a bunch of clocks together in the same room, they will all start to tick at the same rate. Even if you set them somewhat differently, within three to five days, they will all be ticking together. It is normal for us to get in sync with everything around us. If you become in sync with all the people around you who are in judgment, then you create more judgment and limitation of your body.

You have entrained yourself to judgment as if it were real. It's not real. You don't have to do this. Buying other people's judgments is simply a choice you make. Maybe you're like the person who told me, "As a child, everything I created was judged as bad and wrong, and I took that on. Now it doesn't matter what I create, I judge it as wrong." This is an example of entraining yourself with other people's points of view. We all do this. If you grew up with people who were in judgment of their bodies, you learned that you had to be in judgment of your body too. Maybe your parents didn't talk about their judgments of their bodies, but they still had them—and you, the little psychic demon that you are—were aware of it. We entrain ourselves to be in alignment and agreement with other people's judgments of our body, which means you see your body through the judgments and points of view of everybody around you. To whatever degree you entrain with your family or your culture, to that degree you also entrain how you create your body! If you are willing to be ambiguous and move outside everybody else's entrainment, then you get the choice of how you would like to create your body and your life.

A Caucasian woman who lives in South Korea told me that if you aren't a stick figure in Korea (where everyone is thin), you're considered a fatso. A friend who lived on a Pacific island told me that the people there (who are very large) felt sorry for her because she was skinny. Is either of those points of view real? No! They're simply judgments that everyone in those places agreed to. Here is another way of looking at this: You cannot be the effect of anything unless you give it the power to have more value than you, which means you give other people's judgments control over you.

Tool: Who Does This Belong To?

I wanted to find out how not to buy other people's judgments and points of view, so I did an experiment for six months. Every time I had a thought, feeling, or emotion, I asked, **"Who does this belong to?"** At the end of six months, I realized I had no thoughts, feelings, or emotions. I couldn't buy somebody else's point of view as my own, because I knew instantaneously that it belonged to someone else. When you begin to go beyond what everyone else thinks is true, you can begin to create something different for you and your body.

When I talk about this, some people have understood it to mean that because I have no thoughts, feelings, and emotions coming from others, that I am emotionless. That's not true. At my mother's funeral, I cried. I cried because of what I missed. At Christmas time, I cry at every television program and most commercials, because wouldn't it be nice if they were actually true? I cry for what isn't—not for what is. My emotions are the result of what I see missing in the world that would be wonderful to have. I don't cry over the milk I spill.

Tool: Is That Your Point of View?

Start asking your kids questions about their points of view. A friend told me that sometimes her daughter would come home from school and say things that seemed odd.

> My friend would ask her daughter, "Is that your point of view—or is it somebody else's?"
>
> The daughter would say, "Oh, somebody else's."
>
> My friend would say, "So, do you have to buy that as yours?"
>
> The daughter would say, "Uh, no."
>
> The mom would then say, "Okay, cool."

Your kids are way more psychic than you are; that's the reason they chose you as parents. They say, "I'll get all these capacities and abilities by taking these people on as my parents."

You've got to start asking your kids questions. Try asking, **"What are you aware of that you don't want to be aware of?"** Their answers are guaranteed to surprise you. A mother whose kids use Access Consciousness tools told me that one day she asked her daughter what she did in school, and the daughter said, "I was in a fight with someone. I felt angry, and I asked, 'Who does this belong to?' and I realized the girl was angry—but I wasn't, so I just walked away."

I love it when kids use these tools, which is one of the reasons I let them come to Access Consciousness classes for free. They pick up the tools instantaneously and use them right away in all aspects of their life. Three girls recently approached me and asked if they could have a kids' class because the adults were so slow and talked about the same thing forever and never got over it. I said, "Yes, I know."

Winning Bodies, Losing Bodies

Recently I was talking with a woman who said she wanted a relationship. I asked, "What about this person?"

She said, "No, he's a loser."

I mentioned someone else and asked, "What about this person?"

She replied, "He's a loser."

I asked, "What about this guy?"

She said, "Oh yes, he's a winner."

As I listened to her, I thought, "Wait a minute! People also do this winner/loser thing with their bodies." They reach conclusions about what a winning body is. They remember when they had a winning body and when they didn't. They decide what a losing body is. They decide what kind of bodies don't count. Let's say you were born as a girl into a culture that believed only boys were valuable. The body style (female) you had didn't count. You would function from the point of view that your body didn't count.

It's a judgment about whether a body is a winner or a loser and whether it counts. "I wouldn't have sex with him. He's a loser." "I would have sex with her. She's a winner!" These are judgments. You get caught up in judgment about winners or losers, and you lose the capacity to generate or create something that will work for you. Let's say somebody lusts after your body. You become a winner or a loser based on your judgment of whether the person who lusts after you is a winner or a loser. How's that for fun? Your judgment of the person you attract becomes the determining factor for whether your body is a winner or loser—because only if winners lust after you is your body a winner. And if losers lust after your body, then you and your body are losers.

Old/Young

Many of us have the point of view that a losing body is a body that's getting old. Your point of view is that your body goes from being a winner when you're young to being a loser as it gets older. That's pretty funny, actually, because how many young people like their bodies? Very few! Did you like your body when it was young? Or did you think it was a loser even then? Now, of course, you look back and say, "Twenty! That's when I had a winning body!" That's a judgment. It's not about having a winning or a losing body.

When you look at age as a losing proposition, you begin to see your body as not a winning body any longer. When your body doesn't react the way it used to, when you start to get glaucoma or you need glasses, you decide you've got a body that's beginning to lose. That's not what it's about. It's not about winning or losing. It's about having a sense of peace with your body. Once you can have a sense of peace with your body, you can generate or create it any way you wish.

You've got to realize there's nothing wrong, there's nothing right, there's nothing good, there's nothing bad; there is just what is. When you look at your body, do you feel light inside it? Do you love your body just as it is? Or do you judge it? Do you make it feel heavy with everything you think about it?

"I Love You Just the Way You Are"

You may have a body that wishes to be round, firm, and fully packed. I would like you to understand that some people have bodies that want to be big. They want to be heavy. They don't wish to be Skinny Minnies. Not everyone's body is supposed to look like Twiggy's. And not everybody loves skinny bodies. There are some people who love big bodies. Some people like big butts. Other people like tiny breasts. And some like big butts with tiny breasts. There is a preference for every body. There's always somebody who will love your body, but if you don't love it, they can't.

I had a friend who had a large rear end and tiny breasts. She had wispy, non-existent hair, watery blue eyes with no eyelashes, and eyebrows that were snow white. She looked like nothing at all most of the time, except she so loved her body that she would wiggle it up and down and her little breasts would bounce in one direction and her big butt would bounce in another direction. She thought she was just hot as hell—and she had good-looking men dropping at her feet nonstop. Why? Because she *loved* her body! Have you refused to love your body just the way it is? There's a Billy Joel song called *I Love You Just the Way You Are.* You should be singing that song to your body.

Stop judging your body. It's your creation! Why not look at it as the great gift that you created for yourself, and the rest of the world, to see and play with? Why not be happy with it instead of thinking that it's wrong? Right now—enjoy your body. Stop judging it and ask yourself, **"What energy, space, and consciousness can my body and I be that would allow us to enjoy each other totally all the time with total ease?"**

What if you enjoyed your body just as it was?
What if you had peace with your body?

Chapter 5

Vibrational Virtual Realities

Wait a minute. I don't have to create through this reality to get what I want.

I can create my own reality.

People often talk to me about wanting to create a different body. The biggest barrier to doing this is looking for the way to get your body "right." This is something most of us have done. We look at the configuration of our body based on the vibrational virtual realities (VVRs) of this reality. VVRs tell us what everyone else thinks our body (and everything else in our life) is supposed to look like or what is supposed to happen when we get to a certain age.

For your whole life, you've taken on VVRs and looked at yourself through the eyes of everybody else. You don't see through your own eyes. It's like walking around looking at life from a point of view that has nothing to do with you. Pick up a Coke bottle or a water glass with a thick bottom and look through it. Can you see anything clearly? That's what it's like when you look through vibrational virtual realities and try to get clarity on how to create your body or your life. None of what you see is real or true.

As a kid, you came into this reality with no point of view and you watched everybody looking through filters to figure out where they were, what they should do, and how they should be. You thought, "Oh! I see! I need to look through everybody else's eyes to figure out what works here." And pretty soon you were looking at yourself and the world through the green filter or the blue filter or some other filter that has nothing to do with seeing what is. You continuously looked through a reality that was not yours to create your body. But how could it become *your* body when you were looking at it through everyone else's judgments?

Here's an interesting example of creating your body through the vibrational virtual realities of this reality: I talked with a lady from Argentina who said, "It's so strange that women in America have PMS. We don't have PMS in Argentina. Nobody knows about PMS. Nobody knows you're supposed to have it."

How does that work? If you know you're supposed to have PMS, you'll have it. If no one around you has it, and you've never heard of it, you won't have it. How many things have you bought into to make sure you will have everything you are supposed to have, including PMS?

If you accept someone else's standard that it's wrong for your body to be heavy, are you really seeing your body—or are you seeing *judgments* of your body? You're creating your body from the judgments of this vibrational virtual reality.

Have you bought the point of view that a lean and buff body is what everybody is supposed to have? Have you decided that's what your body needs to look like? And have you bought into everyone else's idea of how you're supposed to get that? Those are all vibrational virtual realities.

Do you ever say things such as, "I want to be skinny like I used to be!" You used to be skinny because you were willing to let yourself be skinny. You stayed skinny because you thought you didn't want to grow up—then when you decided you wanted to grow up, you grew up the way everybody else does. You put on some weight. If you're a man over 40, you're not supposed to have a six-pack; you're supposed to have a keg. If you're a woman over 40, your butt is supposed to get fatter every year. We buy those points of view for what reason?

CCCRs

CCCRs are the contribution, the character, the costume, and the role you believe you need to take on to function in this reality. Say you have a female body. You may look at the female bodies around you and say, "Oh, to be a really good female, I need to have large breasts and big hips." If your body doesn't have that, you judge yourself as wrong. If you have a male body, you may look at the male bodies around you and think you need to build your body so you have big muscles. That's the contribution, the character, the costume, and the role you take on. Mostly it's a costume. Your body is primarily the costume that you wear every day so people will know who you are when you walk down the street.

All of those things—the big breasts or the big muscles—are conclusions we reach based on the judgments in play around us. None of those are an actual choice. You take these things on without asking, "What would I like to have as my body?" or "Body, what would you like to look like?" Most of us do not have a clue what we would actually like to choose as our bodies. We decide on the way we want our body to be by looking at magazines, TV, or movies. We say, "That's the body I'd like to have." It may not even be the body we actually wish to have; it may be that's what others have judged to be the ideal body.

When you operate in the vibrational virtual realities of this reality, you always look for what's right about the choices other people are making and the way they're living. You think that something must be right because everybody's doing it or something must be true because everybody's saying it. VVRs lead you to decisions such as "My body is supposed to be voluptuous" or "My body is supposed to be young." You look around to see if you are creating something that looks like what everybody else is creating. You think this is the way to do it right and to get your share of the pie.

Women have said to me, "When I was 30, I thought, 'If only I could be as pretty as I was when I was 15.' Then I got to be 45, and I said, 'If only I could be as pretty as I was when I was 30!'" They look at pictures of themselves when they were 15 and say, "Oh! I didn't look as bad as I felt!" You never notice how you look at the time you are in. You only see yourself through your judgments. You adopt vibrational virtual realities to create an image of who you are in the world, but it doesn't work. It is not really your body that you see, feel, perceive, know, be, or receive. You actually look a whole lot better now than you think you do. The good news is that in fifteen 15 years, you'll look back and see how good you look now!

I've watched different female friends who are a little heavy, and when they finally find a guy they think is way too much fun and start having a great time, they suddenly lose three inches from their hips in four days. How does that work? I've seen people gain weight when they aren't eating anything. What explains these things? It's because we look at our body through judgment-colored glasses. How much of what's going on with your body right now is an alignment and an agreement with some point of view that has been perpetrated on you?

We live from vibrational virtual realities as though there is something correct about them. We think they are real because everybody else aligns and agrees with those points of view. Everything that is out in the world right now is based on an idea that people aligned and agreed with. When you get enough people aligning and agreeing with a point of view, what are you going to create? You are going to create that thing happening, whatever it is! Most of us have spent our lives giving energy to things that we don't actually believe in. We think that if we believe strongly enough, that eventually the thing we hope will occur, will occur. But it doesn't work that way.

This applies to what we call our limitations. It also applies to our belief that we have to learn things: "I have to learn this. I have to study this. I have to know everything about this. If I study hard enough and long enough, I'll get to the point where I can do or be this." And yet there are people who come along that are called idiot savants. They instantly pick things up and do them. How can they do that—and we can't? My point of view is that we are limited by vibrational virtual realities, and they are not.

Generating From Total Awareness

If vibrational virtual realities were based on what's true, then wouldn't everything you have attempted to do have worked instantly? Has it? My guess is you will probably say, "Well, no, it hasn't." That's because in this reality, we create everything only and solely through VVRs. We think we have to go through this reality to find our reality or to find the right answer, in order to get clear on what is appropriate or what's right or how to make things work.

If you're subject to the rules and regulations of the vibrational virtual realities of this reality, can you be the magic you could be with a body? No. If you've made it a priority not to be with your body, not to enjoy embodiment, not to have all the awareness of what it's like to be embodied, then you cannot have the magic that is available when you are truly being you. What if living with your body was a level of magic that can only exist if you're willing to be that magic? Would that mean you could change anything—or that you couldn't? It means you could change anything.

So, What's Real?

If everything out there in front of you is a vibrational virtual reality, then what's real? What's real is your capacity to perceive, know, be, and receive infinitely. Generating from total awareness is different from creating through vibrational virtual realities. What if you could step out of vibrational virtual reality and just be different? What if you could simply have things work based on your own awareness and your own choice? That's the whole idea!

Stirring the Pot

When I work with people, I like to stir the pot. If I stir the pot, you won't be able to burn the bottom of the kettle, and you're going to have a really sweet tasting soup called *YOU*. I like to do these things with humor, because it's not as confrontational. Everything is harder when you're serious. Life is much easier when you're happy and laughing. I don't want anybody to take me seriously, because I get a lot more accomplished when people think I'm funny. I don't confront them about their issue because if I confronted them, they would fight to keep the rightness of their point of view. If I can do it with a little kind sarcasm and a little humor, I can sometimes slip things in around the edge. It's like adding a little spice to the recipe instead of inundating the soup with salt or pepper.

The greatest amount of charge around an issue is released with laughter and not tears. I watch people cry all the time, "Boo-hoo! It's so sad," then five minutes later they're talking about their issue again and in another ten minutes, they're crying once again.

> I say, "Wait a minute! Don't you want to get rid of this?"
>
> They say, "Yes! I want to get rid of it. Take it away from me!"
>
> I say, "Okay, I'm going to take it away!"
>
> They say, "No, you can't!"
>
> I say, "What do you mean I can't?"
>
> They say, "You can't take it away because if you did, I wouldn't know how to be! There would be nothing left of me."
>
> I ask, "So, what makes you think you wouldn't know how to be?"

The problem is that you define yourself by the way other people define themselves. They define their sensitivity based on how much emotional trauma they have. They define their awareness based on how much they can think about things. They define their physical reality based on all the things they're doing in order to be successful. *Doing* becomes the source of *being*. Is any of that really being? Is any of that really awareness? Is any of that really necessary? No!

What would happen if you began to be aware? There would be nothing left of the trauma, drama, upset, and intrigue that you've defined as you. When you perceive, know, be, and receive everything infinitely, you can change in a heartbeat—but instead we lock ourselves into judgments, VVRs, and other points of view as though that's the way to create us. What if you could clear these things? How much freedom would you have? Well, the good news is, you can clear them. There is a clearing process we use in Access Consciousness to destroy and uncreate judgment, VVRs, and other blockages and limitations.

The Clearing Process

Here's how it works: The basis of the universe is energy. Every particle of the universe has energy and consciousness. There is no good energy or bad energy; there is just energy. (It is only your judgment that makes anything good or bad.) Energy is present, mutable, and changeable upon request. It is the substance by which transformation occurs. Everything you say, everything you think, and everything you do generates what occurs in your life. Whatever you choose puts the energy of the universe, the energy of consciousness, into action—and that shows up as your life. This is what your life looks like in this very moment.

Point of Creation, Point of Destruction

Every limitation we have was created by us somewhere throughout all time, space, dimensions, and realities. It involved making a judgment or a decision or taking on a point of view. How and why it was created does not matter, nor does any other part of its story. We only need to know *that* it was created. We call this the point of creation (POC). The point of creation energetically includes the thoughts, feelings, and emotions immediately preceding the decision, judgment, or point of view we took on.

There is also a point of destruction. The point of destruction (POD) is the point where we destroyed our being by taking on a decision or a position that was based on a limited point of view. We literally put ourselves into a destructive universe. The point of destruction, like the point of creation, energetically includes the thoughts, feelings, and emotions immediately preceding the destructive decision.

When you ask a question about a blockage or a limitation, you call up the energy that has you locked into it. You can then destroy and uncreate the blockage or limitation (as well as the thoughts, feelings, and emotions connected to it) with an Access clearing statement. The clearing statement allows you to energetically undo these things so you then have a different choice.

The Clearing Statement

These are the words that make up the clearing statement:

Everything that is, times a godzillion, destroy and uncreate it all. Right and wrong, good and bad, POD and POC, all nine, shorts, boys, and beyonds.

You don't have to understand the clearing statement for it to work, but if you wish to know more about it, there is additional information in the glossary.

With the clearing statement, I am not giving you answers or trying to get you to change your mind. I know that doesn't work. You are the only one who can unlock the points of view that have you trapped. What I am offering here is a tool you can use to change the energy of the points of view that have you locked into unchanging situations.

To use the clearing statement, ask a question designed to bring up the energy of what has you trapped, including all the crap built on top of it or hiding behind it, then say or read the clearing statement to clear the limitation and change it. The more you run the clearing statement, the deeper it goes, and the more layers and levels it can unlock for you.

How Does the Clearing Process Work?

Asking a question brings up an energy, which you will be aware of. Let's use this question:

> *What physical actualization of the terminal and eternal disease of the creation of bodies only and solely through the vibrational virtual realities of this reality do you have that maintains and entrains what you cannot change, choose, and institute as a totally different body?*

It's not necessary to look for an answer to this question. In fact, the answer may not come to you in words. It may come to you as an energy. You may not even cognitively know what the answer to the question is. It doesn't matter how the awareness comes to you. Just ask the question and then clear the energy with the Access clearing statement:

> *Everything that is times a godzillion, will you destroy and uncreate it all? (Say yes here, but only if you truly mean it.) Right and wrong, good and bad, POD and POC, all nine, shorts, boys, and beyonds.*

The clearing statement may seem nonsensically wordy. It is designed to short-circuit your mind so that you can see what choices you have available. If you could work everything out with your logical mind, you would already have everything you desired. Whatever is keeping you from having what you desire is not logical. It's the insane points of view we wish to destroy. The clearing statement is designed to fry every point of view that you have so that you can start to function from your awareness and your knowing. You are an infinite being, and you, as an infinite being, can perceive everything, know everything, be everything, and receive everything. Only your points of view create the limitations that stop that.

Don't make this significant. You're just clearing energy and any points of view, limitations, or judgments you've created. You can use the full clearing statement as I've given it, or you can just say, "POD and POC and all the stuff I read in the book." Try it. It may change your relationship with your body—and everything else in your life. Remember: It's about the energy. Go with the energy of it. You can't do this wrong. You may find that you have a different way of functioning as a result of using the clearing statement.

Only that which you make real becomes that which controls you or owns you.

* * *

Some Additional Processes You Can Do

Everything you've done to make yourself vibrationally attuned to everything that is creating the body that you currently have, will you destroy and uncreate all that? Right and wrong, good and bad, POD and POC, all nine, shorts, boys, and beyonds.

What physical actualization of the terminal and eternal disease of the creation of bodies only and solely through the vibrational virtual realities of this reality do you have that maintains and entrains what you cannot change, choose, and institute as a totally different body? Everything that is times a godzillion, will you destroy and uncreate it all? Right and wrong, good and bad, POD and POC, all nine, shorts, boys, and beyonds.

What physical actualization of the terminal and eternal disease of the creation of muscle solely and only through the VVRs of this reality do you have that maintains and entrains what you cannot change, choose, and institute as a lean and buff body? Everything that is times a godzillion, will you destroy and uncreate it all? Right and wrong, good and bad, POD and POC, all nine, shorts, boys, and beyonds.

What physical actualization of the terminal and eternal disease of the CCCRs for body building do you have that maintains and entrains everything you cannot change or alter in and as your body and your life? Everything that is times a godzillion, will you destroy and uncreate it all? Right and wrong, good and bad, POD and POC, all nine, shorts, boys, and beyonds.

What physical actualization of the terminal and eternal disease of the creation of reality only and solely through the vibrational virtual realities of this reality do you have that maintains and entrains what you cannot change, choose, and institute as a totally different reality of your own? Everything that is times a godzillion, will you destroy and uncreate it all? Right and wrong, good and bad, POD and POC, all nine, shorts, boys, and beyonds.

What physical actualization of the terminal and eternal disease of the creation of your sexual reality only and solely through the vibrational virtual realities of this reality do you have that maintains and entrains what you cannot change, choose, and institute as a totally different sexual reality? Everything that is times a godzillion, will you destroy and uncreate it all? Right and wrong, good and bad, POD and POC, all nine, shorts, boys, and beyonds.

What physical actualization of the terminal and eternal disease of the creation of money only and solely through the vibrational virtual realities of this reality do you have that maintain and entrains what you cannot change, choose, and institute as a totally different financial reality? Everything that is times a godzillion, will you destroy and uncreate it all? Right and wrong, good and bad, POD and POC, all nine, shorts, boys, and beyonds.

Note: You can do the processes as they are given throughout the book using the words you and your—and answering yes to the question, "Will you destroy and uncreate it?". Or if you prefer, you can change the wording so you are addressing the questions to yourself using I and my—and then simply say "destroy and uncreate it." Either way works.

Chapter 6

Creating Something Different With Your Body

No matter what, this body is my creation!
Now, am I happy with this creation or would I like to create something different?

Throughout my life, I always wanted to look like the Incredible Hulk. I wanted big, well-defined muscles—lots of them—but I could never make that happen. I'd go to the gym to work out, but I could never build big muscles. Instead I would get lean and skinny. This was very annoying, since I had a fixed idea about how I wanted to look. The thing is, it was somebody else's standard. It wasn't mine—and it certainly wasn't my body's.

Then, when I was about 60, I got to the point where I was wearing size 38 pants—and growing. I was in the process of becoming an endomorph, a little fat man, and I was not happy about that. I looked at myself and said, "This is not acceptable. I am not interested in this. This does not work for me!"

I finally asked my body what *it* wanted to look like. One day about six months later, I was watching TV and I saw a guy who had a long, lean body with well-defined muscles. It was a swimmer's body. My body said, "There! That's what I want to look like!" It wanted to be an ectomorph; a lean, skinny guy. I said, "*That's* what you want to look like? We can't look like that! We're over 60 and our hips are too big (because everyone knows that when you're over 60, your hips are supposed to spread and things happen that keep you from moving correctly).

> Then I said, "Well, okay, if you want to look like that, I'll do whatever it takes to make that happen."
>
> About a week later, Dain said, "Let's go to the beach and play Frisbee."
>
> I said, "Okay," and we drove to the beach.

We were running in the sand, and all of a sudden my hips went crack-crack-crack and they suddenly became two inches thinner. I had to be willing to let go of my fixed point of view that because I was 60, I couldn't have that occur. You've got to let go of whatever point of view you have that is creating a conflict between you and your body.

Whatever size your body is, whatever shape it is, if you ask it what it wants to look like and then work with it, it will create itself in a different way. But we don't do that. We decide what we want our body to look like and then we impose that image on it. We make a decision and a judgment about the way it should look. But what if that's not what our body wants to look like?

It's not about the body *you* would like to have, because the body you'd like to have is based on judgments, which are usually created by other people's points of view of how it's supposed to look and be. Your body knows what it wants to look like. It has its own point of view. Do you ever ask it or give it a choice? For most of us, the answer is no. You've got to ask the body!

- *Body, what would you like to look like?*
- *What would you like to feel like?*
- *What would you like to dress like?*
- *What would you like to function as?*

If your body wishes to look like something you consider improbable, say it wants to be long and lean and it is currently anything but that, or say it wants to be like the body you had 10 years ago, then you have to ask:

- *What would it take to create a body like that?*
- *What would we have to be, do, have, create, or generate to generate our body more like that?*

You Created Your Body

Are you willing to own that you created your body exactly as it is? And that it is a brilliant creation? Or do you judge it as wrong? Each of us has a body that is beautiful in ways we don't want to know. We're not willing to own its beauty. The one thing we are always willing to own is the wrongness of our body. We will own the wrongness of our body's appearance or its weight or its lack of energy. We will make those wrongnesses real, important, and true for us. We're willing to own the wrongness of everything we do and everything we are. We are even willing to own the wrongness of our body's beauty. But we are not willing to own the greatness of our body.

You've got to get that you created embodiment. Embodiment is not just your physical form; it's this whole reality. Everything you experience in this reality is part of what you created. Once you acknowledge that, you can ask, **"Is that something I want to continue to create?"**

Your body may not be everything you would like it to be right now, but you created it. So somewhere, it is correct. It's not wrong. Choose to feel grateful for your body exactly as you've created it and keep being grateful until you have the peace, relaxation, and calm that you and your body truly desire.

When you go into, "I don't like my body, I don't like the way it looks," you're invalidating what you have created. You're judging your creation. Don't judge your creations. Don't invalidate your body. Don't compare it to other bodies. Every time you look at your body and start to judge it, immediately stop judging and ask, **"What is brilliant about this creation?"**

> *Everything you've done to make your body wrong, when it's really right because it has created itself just the way you've asked, everything that is times a godzillion, will you destroy and uncreate it all? Right and wrong, good and bad, POD and POC, all nine, shorts, boys, and beyonds.*

Creating Something Different

In order to create something totally different with your body, you've got to acknowledge that you created your body in the first place. Until you acknowledge that you are the creator, nothing can change. This doesn't apply just to your body; it applies to your money, your work, your relationships, and everything else in your life. Come out of the place where you have a sense that you didn't create something (whether it's your body or anything else) and go into the place where you realize you created it. If you don't acknowledge that you created it, you can't change it. Even if you can't come out of judging it, you can at least acknowledge that you created it: "Look at this thing I've created. Wow, if I can create something this bad, imagine what I could create if I went in a different direction!"

> *How many points of view are you using to create the body you're not happy with? Oops! Everything that is times a godzillion, will you destroy and uncreate it all? Right and wrong, good and bad, POD and POC, all nine, shorts, boys, and beyonds.*

> Someone said to me, "It seems like it would take a lot of courage to be so different that you no longer bought into judgment."
>
> I said, "It's not so much that it takes courage; it takes a willingness to recognize that you create everything. Everything you think, everything you be,[vii] everything you do is your creation. Whatever occurs in your life is what you created."

Change can occur when you come out of believing you didn't create your life and you go into the place where you realize: "I created this. No matter what it is, this is my creation! Now, am I happy with this creation—or would I like

vii See the Glossary for a note on the use of the word *be*.

to have something different?" When you start to own that, you begin to own what is truly possible in your life. You start to be capable of creating change in the places you wish to create a change. It's: "Okay, I'm the one who created this. So, now what would I like to create?" It's not: "What's wrong with me that I can't create this?"

I create everything.

Everything I think, everything I be, everything I do, is my creation.

Whatever occurs in my life is what I have created.

You Don't Need to Know the How or the Why

The only reason you can't change your body into something different is because you created it and then you bought the lie that you didn't create it. You can begin to choose differently by being grateful for what you have done and by seeing the brilliance of your creation. Feeling gratitude leads to peace, relaxation, and calmness. This is the key. It's: "Wow, I am so glad I created this body!" You can even be grateful for the pain or discomfort in your body. "Wow, I've created this pain. How cool am I? Was that a good choice? No, it wasn't. Okay, what's next? What do I want to create now?"

Oftentimes when I talk with people about changing their body, they want to look at the *how* or the *why* of their current body situation. I tell them, "You don't need to know the *how* or the *why* of it. It's just that you keep choosing what you have for some reason that you don't remember. Don't bother trying to figure out why you created it the way you did. Just acknowledge that you did it."

Here's an example. My desk used to be covered in tall stacks of paper. You couldn't see the desk for all the paper that was on it. I hated the fact that I wouldn't file it and couldn't seem to do anything with it. One day I finally said, "Wait a minute! I can't possibly hate this! Obviously I love it—because I keep creating it! I love creating this mess. I love creating stacks of paper. I love having all this stuff on top of my desk. Now, what would I like to change? Or do I want to do anything different? Do I want to change it?"

This is what you have to do as well. It's not: "I created it and now I have to figure out why I created it or else I can't uncreate it. I've got to know how or why I do this, because if I don't know the *how* or the *why*, then I can't undo it." That's a lie you are buying!

The real *why* in life is simply *that* you did it. That's the only thing you have to know. "I did this—and if I created this what else can I create?" You simply choose again. It's not: "The reason I'm heavy is because I'm protecting myself. The reason I'm heavy is because I eat too much. The reason I'm heavy is because I have a bad metabolism." None of those reasons are why you created the weight. You created it because it was a brilliant idea at the time. The times have now changed, and it may not be the same brilliant idea.

You Are the Change Agent for Your Body

You may believe change can occur—but you may think it can't occur unless you do the "right" thing. You may think that changing your body is about moving it the right way or eating the right foods or doing some other right thing—but those are not the source of change. You are the source of change for your body! *You* are the change agent for your body.

You're the potency and the catalyst that changes anything and everything. All you have to do is change your point of view. You don't have to change your diet. You don't have to change your clothes. You don't even have to change your underwear. You just have to change your point of view! Your points of view are the long johns you have been wearing for the past two billion years, and they are kind of smelly right now. You could at least take them off and wash them before you put them back on.

Exercise vs. Movement

If you're trying to get a body that's more lean and muscled, then you need a willingness to do whatever your body wants. When I ask my body what it wants to do, and it says, "Go do _____," I go do it, and everything suddenly looks better in my body. Why does everything look better in my body? Because I did what my body told me to do!

When you look through the vibrational virtual realities of this reality, all you hear is: "You have to work out, you have to lift weights, you have to do *x*, *y*, and *z*. You can't do it this way. You can't do it that way." I've had people say, "You can't build muscle in twenty minutes," but I've had the experience of doing the Access Consciousness process MTVSS[viii] while working out—and I built muscle in twenty minutes, so that can't be correct. There has to be some lie we're buying with the VVRs of this reality that maintains and entrains what we cannot change, choose, and institute as a lean and buff body.

Ask your body what it wants to do. The body likes to move, but it doesn't like to exercise, because it hears *ex-or-cise*, which means you're going to take the being out of the body, and it doesn't want the being to leave. It likes the being. When you try to make your body exercise, you're going against its basic point of view—and when you try to make it sedentary you're also going against its basic point of view. Bodies like to move; they don't like to be stationary.

There's a lot of fun in movement. What kind of movement is fun for you and your body? For some people, dancing is fun; for other people, walking is fun; for others, riding horses is fun. Because the body likes movement, you need to ask, "Body, what movement would you like today?" It may desire to dance or it may desire to go for a run or it may desire to have a massage. Is that exercise? No, but it is movement.

viii Information about how to do MTVSS is in the Glossary.

I used to go to the gym, and I finally got to the point where I couldn't go any more. It was hard on me to hear the bodies screaming, "Please make this person stop!" I watched people with perfect bodies working out like crazy in front of the mirror, saying "I've got to do more! I've got to do more!" and their bodies were screaming, "Enough! I'm over this. I can't stand this! It hurts!" People were hurting their bodies because they had taken on the point of view of "no pain, no gain" rather than asking, "Body, what do you need?"

These people had beautiful bodies, but they were judging every single inch of them as wrong. Were they actually looking at their bodies? No, they were looking at their *judgments* of their bodies. It's manic insanity.

> After I learned to ask my body questions, I would go to the gym to work out, and I would ask, "Okay body, which machine do you want to work out on?"
>
> My body would say, "That one."
>
> I'd say, "That one's out of order."
>
> My body would say, "Yeah, I know."

I would ask my body what it wanted to do, and that's what I'd do. And I would get better results in twenty minutes of doing whatever my body wanted to do than I would get out of an hour and a half of working out in the conventional way. This is not the way you're supposed to work out at the gym—but it's what my body wanted, and that's what worked for us.

What physical actualization of the terminal, eternal, and infectious disease of never fully embodying the change you can truly be do you have that maintains and entrains what you cannot change, choose, and institute as your body? Everything that is times a godzillion, will you destroy and uncreate it all? Right and wrong, good and bad, POD and POC, all nine, shorts, boys, and beyonds.

It's Not About What Worked in the Past

Sometimes when people want to change something in their life or their body, they are drawn to use what worked for them in the past. They say things like, "It has always worked for me to eat well" or "It has always worked for me to ____." This is called referencing the past. We look at something we did in the past that seemed to work and we think, "Oh, that's what I should do." No! That worked *then*, this is *now*.

What's different now that you're not acknowledging? Let's say you felt powerless as a kid and therefore you had a little body that was slim and trim. You decided you wanted to grow up and to be big and powerful. Have you gotten big enough to be powerful yet? Or do you still think you're puny in some way—and that's what's creating the body you're not happy with? Do you still think you're powerless over creating a body? Instead of looking to be what you were in the past, what if you just got happy with your creation and asked it to create itself as something different?

> *Everything you decided in the past as a creation of your body, will you now please destroy and uncreate it all? Right and wrong, good and bad, POD and POC, all nine, shorts, boys, and beyonds.*

Please enjoy your sweet body. I enjoy your body every chance I get to see it.

I love the fact that you are all different sizes and shapes and all different people.

And you should too.

* * *

Additional Processes You Can Do

How many lies have you locked into reality about your body that are creating it exactly the way it should not be, would not be, and would not choose to be if you would let it be what it would like to be? Everything that is times a godzillion, will you destroy and uncreate it all? Right and wrong, good and bad, POD and POC, all nine, shorts, boys, and beyonds.

Have you decided you can't change your body? Have you concluded you can't change it because you're over 30 or you're over 40—and it's downhill from here? Have you made a decision, a judgment, a computation, or a conclusion that you will never be able to change your body? Everything that is times a godzillion, will you destroy and uncreate it all? Right and wrong, good and bad, POD and POC, all nine, shorts, boys, and beyonds.

What energy can you be that you are refusing to be? Everything that doesn't allow that to show up times a godzillion, will you destroy and uncreate it all? Right and wrong, good and bad, POD and POC, all nine, shorts, boys, and beyonds.

What energy can you and your body be? Everything that doesn't allow that to show up times a godzillion, will you destroy and uncreate it all? Right and wrong, good and bad, POD and POC, all nine, shorts, boys, and beyonds.

What energy, space, and consciousness can you and your body be that would allow you to be and appear exactly as you would like to be and appear? Everything that doesn't allow that to show up times a godzillion, will you destroy and uncreate it all? Right and wrong, good and bad, POD and POC, all nine, shorts, boys, and beyonds.

Chapter 7

Food And Eating

Who needs food—you or your body?
The truth is that neither of you need food.

Sometimes people tell me they need to be more mindful of things; for example, they'll say, "I need to be more mindful when I work with horses" or "I need to be more mindful of my body."

I say, "You don't have to be mindful; you just have to be energetically connected." Trying to be mindful means you have to think about it, you have to figure it out, you have to put attention on it. This is very different from being aware of the energy. When you start to be more aware of the energy with horses, dogs, and cats; with your body; and with other people too, you access a level of communication that is far greater than any kind of verbal communication. Your ears only hear the limitations. Your awareness hears the possibilities.

Recently we were doing a Conscious Horse, Conscious Rider Clinic. One of the horses we were working with kept running away from its owner. I was across the pasture from it, and I energetically said, "Stop." It looked at me and went, "Oh!" and stopped in its tracks. It stood there until I walked up to it and put a halter on it.

> The horse's owner said, "How did you do that? He's always running away from me."
>
> I said, "I put an energy there that allowed the horse to know he is mine, and he is not allowed to do anything I don't want him to do."

Horses communicate telepathically. So do people and so do bodies. We try not to communicate telepathically; instead we do verbal diarrhea as though people are going to understand us. Get over it. People aren't going to understand your verbal diarrhea. How often do you just *know* something and it always works out? How often do you try to *explain* something to someone and the person says, "I don't understand what you're talking about"?

The reality is every molecule in the world communicates with us. If we would molecularly communicate with all things (including our bodies) and allow ourselves to be aware, we would receive the information they give us and would not need to do 90 percent of the things we do—including the way we eat.

Food

It's great fun to go to big box stores like Costco or Walmart and buy huge quantities of food. People fill up two carts full of groceries and waddle out of the place. You're waddling if you have two carts of food—because you're trying to eat all of that stuff so you don't waste the money you spent on it.

Who needs food—you or your body? The truth is that neither of you need food. That's an interesting point of view, isn't it? What if you didn't need food at all? What if eating food was just a choice?

Bodies want energy; they don't want food, and people think food will give their body the energy it desires. But food does not give you energy. It actually makes you soporific; it makes you want to sleep. Have you ever noticed that you eat and then you want to take a nap? Digesting food uses all the energy of your body. Large amounts of food eliminate your capacity to generate and create and put you into a place where you need to sleep in order to have a sense of connection with your body. In southern Europe, for example, everything's closed after lunch for several hours. If you show up at a restaurant in Italy after two o'clock, you can't find anything to eat. They're closed. Everybody's taking a nap because they had a big lunch.

The reality is that food should be like a homeopathic dose of medicine for releasing energy in your body. Small amounts of food can give you the energy your body needs. Large amounts of food require more energy to digest than you receive from eating it in the first place.

Do You Really Need to Eat?

The mitochondria in our cells is the power producer. They convert energy into forms that are usable by the cell. Each person has enough energy in the mitochondria of their cells to run a city the size of Chicago for three months. If you have that kind of energy in your body, what is it that makes you think you have to eat to get energy?

Do you really need to eat? Or is that a point of view you've taken on? Before your next meal, ask your body if it would like to eat. If it doesn't want to eat, ask if it wants something to drink. Or does it want to go for a walk?

If it wants to eat, ask it what it would like to eat and get that. Eat the first three bites of each thing on your plate in total consciousness. This means don't talk to the people you're eating with. Savor each morsel as you put it in your mouth and experience how it reacts on every taste bud in the different locations on your tongue. Each taste bud acts at a different level of sensation depending on what's in the item you're eating. Let yourself notice where the different taste buds activate according to sweet and sour and different flavors so that food becomes a sensuous experience, not a filling experience.

After eating the first three bites of each thing on your plate, continue to eat very slowly. The moment your food begins to taste like cardboard, stop eating. How many bites will that be? About nine. Your body is telling you that is all it needs to open the doors to massive amounts of energy for you. Everything else is stored in the fat cells of your body.

When you do this, you will begin to see what is occurring in your body. It's about getting connected to the skin you're in. The result is that you will be totally present with your body in a new way. The moment the food doesn't taste fabulous, *stop eating*. Your body is telling you that's all it requires. It's about becoming aware of what your body needs. We eat 90 percent more than we actually need because we have been taught to clean our plates. We have been taught to eat three balanced meals every day; we've been taught all kinds of things that have nothing to do with allowing our body to choose for itself.

> One woman who tried this said that after each bite she would ask her body, "Okay, are you finished?"
>
> It would say, "No, a little more," and she'd take another bite.
>
> Then she would ask, "How about now?"
>
> Again her body would say, "Just a little more."
>
> She would take one more bite, and her body would say, "I don't think you want this any more."
>
> She would reply, "No, we don't."

When you function in this way, you start to recognize, "This is how I can know what my body's point of view is." You eat until your body suddenly says, "Bleah," and then you don't eat any more. You drink the same way. When I have a glass of wine, the first several sips will taste great and then all of a sudden, the next sip will taste like vinegar. That's my body saying, "Okay, that's enough." It does not desire any more. If you practice this, you will get to the place where you're not overeating, and your body will not create burps and farts as a way of punishing you. (Your body uses burps and farts as a punishment system when you don't listen.)

This is not meant to be a diet. It's a new perspective. You may not lose an ounce doing this, but you will get to the point where you can actually hear your body. You'll discover what it likes, what it requires, and where to take it at the right moment. You will have a lot more fun. I guarantee you that.

Hunger

Your body actually likes the feeling of being hungry. What if a hungry body was actually a healthy body—and not an unhealthy body? "I'm hungry" is a fixed point of view. When your body feels spacious, you may misidentify that spacious feeling as hunger. You may say, "I'm hungry" rather than "I feel empty." But what if your body is not hungry? What if it's just feeling space? Bodies like to feel space. They don't like to feel full. If you don't believe me, remember your last Christmas dinner. How did you feel afterward? Most people sit around groaning and asking, "Why did I do it?" What if hunger keeps the body in a state of question? What if filling it up creates an answer?

Someone told me, "The idea of asking my body questions about what it requires is such a gift. When I feel empty, I often get agitated, and I decide that I need to eat something so I can calm down—but I don't know what my body wants to eat. When I ask questions, I discover there's nothing it wants to eat."

I've been asking my body forever what it wants to eat, and as a result, I often eat once a day, no more. If I eat twice a day, it's pretty much a miracle. If I feel hungry, I ask, **"Body, are you hungry—or do you just feel the space you wish to be?"** My body likes to be hungry. It likes to feel space. It doesn't like to feel heavy.

I invite you to change your perspective about hunger and other feelings that you get. When your body needs something, it tries to give you information in the form of a feeling. Actually, *feeling* isn't the best word to describe this. Feelings are not really feelings. They're *senses*. You're sensing things. You can ask, **"What am I sensing?"** Does a so-called feeling mean you're hungry? Not necessarily. Maybe you're having an awareness of something else. When you immediately identify feelings as hunger or pain, you assume a point of view that may be very different from what your body is telling you. Don't assume a feeling means you need to eat! Instead of naming what you feel or assigning some sort of label to it like "hungry," ask a question. What if your body is crying out to go for a walk, and you're thinking you're hungry? If you don't assume you need to eat, you can discover what your body actually requires.

A woman recently told me, "After I eat, I often feel like I'm popping out of my clothes. I haven't eaten that much; I just feel bloated and uncomfortable."

I asked, "Did you ask your body if it wanted to eat at all?"

She said, "No."

I said, "Well, you might try that."

Often I will feel a rumbling in my tummy and I will think, "I'm hungry." But then I ask, "Body, are you hungry?" and it says, *no*. Sometimes I go to the refrigerator anyway and ask, "Is there anything you want to eat in here?" and it says, *no*. So I ask, "Okay do you want some water?" and it says, *yes*. All it wanted was water, but I thought I was hungry.

People have had so many lifetimes in which famine was "real" that even when there is an abundance of food, they continue to eat instead of looking at what's happening for them in the present. It's very hard to starve to death in most countries in the world right now. You have to work hard at it, because there is so much excess everywhere. If we believe there is such a thing as famine, we buy into the idea that we'd better eat now, because we may not be able to eat tomorrow. That's pretty much not true in most Western societies, and in many so-called Third World countries, there always seems to be enough food.

How much of filling your body up is an answer to the assumption that hunger or feeling hungry is wrong and that famine is real? All of it, some of it, or more than all of it? Everything that is times a godzillion, will you destroy and uncreate it all please? Right and wrong, good and bad, POD and POC, all nine, shorts, boys, and beyonds.

"I Love to Eat Well"

When I talked about eating three bites of everything on your plate with a friend, she said, "That wouldn't work for me because I love to eat well."

I asked, "What does 'I love to eat well' have to do with your body? 'I love to eat well.' Is that a truth or is that an entrainment? It's entrainment. It doesn't have anything to do with listening to your body!"

I asked her, "Which do you love more, sex or food?"

She laughed and said, "Sex is more satisfying, but food is more available."

Every time you think you would like some food, I invite you to see what happens if you masturbate instead. See which one (sex or food) you choose under those conditions! What if every time you had a thought about eating, you had sex instead?

The feeling of hunger is actually a way to sharpen your awareness. Do you realize that the more you satiate your hunger, the more of your awareness you turn off? Have you ever noticed that when you eat beyond what your body requires that your awareness and your senses become dulled and that your desire to have sex is diminished?

There is, of course, a point at which you need to eat. Your body requires food, but if you start to pay attention to what your body desires, you have the opportunity to function in a way that creates and generates more awareness for you.

Please pay attention to that. When you feel hungry, instead of asking, "How do I fill my hunger?" ask:

- *Body, what awareness are you giving me?*
- *What do you require or desire?*

Tasting Food

What if you actually received the incredible elegance of one bite of food? One of the reasons I suggest you eat the things on your plate only as long as they taste great is that it will give you a sense of the pleasure of food. It will also introduce you to sensory aestheticism. Your body should be a sensory aesthetic organ.

Years ago when I was married, I would buy a two-pound box of chocolates and I would eat one piece a day. My ex-wife would find them (because I hid them from her) and she'd eat half the box in a single sitting. Do you really enjoy something when you do that? Or would you enjoy it more if you did something different?

Tool: I Wonder What This Is Going to Taste Like

When someone says, "chocolate cake" or "lemon pie" do you instantaneously respond with a comment like, "Mmm, that tastes good!" Most of us do this. We've decided or judged that certain things taste good or bad, and then we don't have to be aware of how they actually taste. I like to invite people to live in the question rather than operating from past decisions, judgments, and computations.

Every time you sit down to eat, act as though you've never before tasted any of the food in front of you. Before you take a bite of that food, say; **"I wonder what this is going to taste like?"**If you do this, you will start tasting food in the present moment instead of referring to the past. This will put you into the question about what you are ingesting instead of sending you into the answer of "I like this" or "I don't like this."

I used to like marshmallow cookies with chocolate over them. I thought they were the most wonderful cookies in the world—then I got fed so many of them at Access functions that I can't stand them anymore. Now when I look at one of them, I go, "Puke." Or is that my body that's going "Puke"? It's my body. I can't override it any more. The more I become aware of what my body desires, the less I can override it.

I hope you will use these tools so you can get to the point where you won't override your body or try to force it to eat what you've decided you like rather than asking it:

- *What would you like to eat?*
- *What would be fun for you to eat?*
- *What's this going to taste like?*

Children and Eating

If you have children, recognize that kids like to graze. They're little animals; they're like horses. They want to graze on things throughout the day. Requiring them to eat three meals is a mistake.

> Ask your kids, "What would your body like to eat?" and then give it to them.
>
> A lady in Texas called me and said, "I ask my son what his body wants to eat, and he always says that it wants ice cream. He says his body wants to eat ice cream for breakfast. It wants ice cream at ten o'clock. It wants ice cream for lunch. I can tell this a lie. What should I do?"
>
> I said, "Keep letting him choose."

She did, and the boy chose ice cream at two o'clock, ice cream at five o'clock, and ice cream at nine o'clock before he went to bed. Then he puked all night long.

> She asked him, "Truth, did your body really want ice cream?"
>
> He said, "No, it didn't really want ice cream, but I thought I could get away with it."

She said, "Okay."

The mother continues to ask her son what his body would like to eat, and since then, he has not gone against what his body really wants. A cool lesson.

Tool: In a Restaurant

Here is something you can try when you go out to eat: Whenever you are eating in a restaurant, open the menu then close your eyes and ask your body to show you what it wants to eat. Open your eyes and they will instantaneously fall on what your body desires. This might be something you've decided you don't like. You might say, "Oh no, I don't like that." At this point, you have a choice. You can order that item anyway, or you can repeat the exercise and ask again.

If you choose to repeat the exercise, know that eventually your body will bypass you. Even if you order what you wish to have, the waiter will bring you food you didn't order. Your body spoke directly to the waiter's body and he brought you what your body asked for. Please be kind to the poor waiter. Eat whatever he brings you and leave him a nice tip. You may find that it tastes better than anything you thought was possible.

After this happens ten or twelve times, you may begin to realize that your body is talking to you, and you may start to trust it a little more. It may take some time for you to develop trust in your body, however, because you have never trusted it before. Your body is your best friend. If you're not trusting your body, you're not trusting you, and you're not trusting that you and your body are best friends.

How much energy are you using not to be best friends with your body? A lot, a little, or megatons beyond megatons beyond megatons? Everything that is times a godzillion, will you destroy and uncreate it all? Right and wrong, good and bad, POD and POC, all nine, shorts, boys, and beyonds.

Tool: At a Dinner Party

Sometimes you might be in a situation where you can't eat what your body would like. Say, for example, you're at a dinner party and they're serving something your body doesn't wish to eat. What can you do? Donnielle approaches it this way: "You're in communion with your body. Talk to it! See what can happen. If I'm at a dinner party where they're serving Italian food and my body doesn't want Italian food, I'll ask it, **"Body, what would it take for us to enjoy this food, digest it, and have no problem with it? What would it take for you utilize the nutritional value and glean whatever you need to from it?"** My body will say, 'Okay,' and be fine with it."

Tool: In a Grocery Store

When you go into a grocery store, ask, **"Body, is there anything here you want to eat?"** If the answer is *no*, leave. If you're married, you can ask, **"Is there anything here my partner's body would like to eat?"** Oftentimes your body doesn't actually wish to eat, but you go to the store in order to feed somebody else's body.

> *How much of what you're eating is you feeding somebody else's body? A lot? A little? Or megatons? Oops. Everything you've done to feed other people's bodies by eating through your body, times a godzillion, will you destroy and uncreate it all? Right and wrong, good and bad, POD and POC, all nine, shorts, boys, and beyonds.*

Planning Meals and Shopping

Do you plan what you're going to eat a week ahead of time? How much of planning what you are going to eat is actually a way of destroying trust in your body? People try to plan out their meals with a fixed point of view about what they're supposed to be eating or what they like to eat. They are not being aware of what their body desires to eat.

It was interesting for me to see that in New York City, they don't have big supermarkets—they have smaller stores in each neighborhood. Most people don't have giant subzero refrigerators and lots of cupboards or storage space, so they can't stock up on huge quantities of food. They have to stop at the store every day or so, and they tend to look at what their body wants. That's where I learned to be more present with my body when I went to the store. I couldn't plan what I was going to eat in the coming week. I just bought enough for this meal and one or two others. I had to be aware of what I could actually use and eat. I would ask my body, **"What are you going to want to eat in the next couple of days?"** It would say, "Oh, that fruit looks good!" or "That broccoli would be nice."

You may wish to start buying smaller amounts of food and shopping more often. People have told me that when they shop daily, they—and their families—have slimmer bodies.

Tool: Muscle Testing

Before I put any kind of substance—a vitamin, a supplement, a medicine, or an herb—in my body, I do muscle testing. You can do this with food as well. I hold the substance in front of my solar plexus and I stand with my heels and my toes together. I ask, **"Body, do you want to ingest this?"**

If my body leans forward, it's a yes. If it leans backward, it's a *no.* If it goes side to side, I know I'm asking the wrong question, so I'll try additional questions such as, **"Do you want to ingest this later? Do you want to ingest this tomorrow?"**

I know a guy in Australia who was having "blood pressure" problems so he went to the doctor, who sent him home with some pills.

> He called me and said, "I just muscle tested the pills to see whether my body wants them, and I got thrown

> backward across the room. My body does not want to take these pills. What should I do?"
>
> I said, "Go to a different doctor and find out what's really going on. Obviously, your body doesn't want the pills you have. It wants something else, and you've got to find out what the something else is."

He went to another doctor and discovered that he did not have high blood pressure at all. He required surgery to put in a shunt that would open up the blood vessels in his heart. He could have died if he had taken the pills the first doctor prescribed. The moral of this story is: Your body knows what it needs. Trust it!

Absorbing Nutrients

At one point awhile ago, I was feeling tired, and I thought, "Oh gosh, I must need some vitamins," so I went to the vitamin store. I was standing in the vitamin section, muscle testing every vitamin on the shelf, and my body was saying, *no, no, no, no, no.* So I walked out of the store with no vitamins, feeling high as a kite.

> I asked, "Body, did you just absorb all the vitamins you needed out of those bottles?"
>
> It said, "Yeah."

Now I just walk through the vitamin section and I tell my body, "Take everything you need, Body." Vitamins are an energy. You don't even have to open the bottle to get the energy. The energy is there, exuding through the plastic. Many people would say the bottles are a solid that nothing passes through. Is that true? No, that's a lie. Is glass something solid that nothing can pass through? No, the molecules just move more slowly through things we've defined as solid. They aren't actually solid.

Go for a Walk in the Woods

If you want to experience what it's like to absorb the nutrients you need, go for a walk in the woods and ask your body to take everything it needs from nature. Have you ever noticed that when you go for a long walk in the woods, you come back feeling energized and excited? Your body feels really good, and you say, "Wow, that was such a great walk!" It wasn't just a great walk; it was a great communion with all the molecular structures around you and a great assimilation by your body of everything it needed. If you start to notice that your body needs healing, go for a walk and ask it to take whatever it needs from nature. It's amazing how quickly that can occur.

Is your body made of energy—or is it made of a molecular structure that has no ability to receive? It's made of energy! Are you creating your body as a molecular structure that can't receive anything? Oops. That's why you have to feed it—because it can't receive. It actually *can* receive, but you won't let it. Why won't you let it? Because if you did, you'd have to be different. And if you were different, you wouldn't be normal. And if you weren't normal, then you couldn't sit down to dinner with people and talk about idiotic things for hours at a time.

Would You Like Something Sweet?

When you'd like something sweet, go into a bakery. Stand there for a few minutes, inhale deeply, and then ask your body, "Are you hungry?" It will say, "No, I just got all the sugar I needed." You just breathed in the molecular structure of everything that sugar provides for your body.

When You're Traveling

I have a friend who travels a great deal. When she's on a plane and her throat starts to feel scratchy, she says to her body, "Hey Body, are we flying over an area where you could pull the energies from herbs or anything else that would assist you in not picking up whatever is circulating in the air?" Then her scratchy throat (or whatever it is) usually goes away, immediately. Try it. It may work for you too.

Preparing Food

Have you ever prepared a dinner, and by the time you're finished cooking, you didn't want to eat? Why didn't you want to eat? You absorbed everything that the food was going to provide. You weren't hungry because you got everything that was going to be served in the meal just by cooking it. If you get how incredibly beautiful and orgasmic your body is, you will see that it will take in everything it needs from just the process of cooking food for others.

Let Your Body Have Control Over Itself

As a kid, were you asked what you wanted or were you told what you had to eat, when you had to go to bed, and when you had to get up? Were you told when you had to go outside and when you had to come in? This causes us to look for an outside source that tells us what to do with our body instead of recognizing that our body knows what to do for itself.

Some people like to keep a food diary to become more aware of what they're eating. You can certainly do this if you wish, but it's really about asking your body what it wants to eat, rather than trying to create a diary about the food you consumed. Keeping a food diary can become a way to attempt to control what you do. I don't want you to control your body. I want you to allow your body to have control over itself. This is a very different point of view. Your body knows what it requires and desires. Ask it!

Eat More! Eat More! Eat More!

People often tell me that as children, they were highly energetic, skinny, and healthy—and they didn't wish to eat. Their family would force them to eat. They would say things like, "Eat! You need to put some meat on your bones" or "If you don't eat, the wind is going to blow you away." That's what they told me.

Are you still trying to put meat on your bones? Are you still trying to grow a big, nice, healthy body? Everything that is times a godzillion, will you destroy and uncreate it all? Right and wrong, good and bad, POD and POC, all nine, shorts, boys, and beyonds.

When you were a kid, were you told that you needed to clean your plate because of the starving children in China? I was. I got in such trouble when I said, "Well, can't we send my Brussels sprouts to them?"

Then there is all the cultural and family entrainment around eating. Most of us were entrained to eat a certain way: You must eat protein, you must eat carbohydrates, you must eat fruit, and you must eat vegetables. You must eat mashed potatoes and gravy for dinner. If you're Italian, you must eat pasta. If you're from the Midwest, you probably have a family that insists you eat three times a day. In my family we had to eat Jell-O salad, green salad, a second Jell-O salad, a third Jell-O salad, and ambrosia. Your family feeds you because that's called love.

You may notice that you have no idea what your reality around eating is. You may be validating other people's realities by the food you choose to eat. When you start to eat or you think about eating something, ask, **"Is this my reality or someone else's?"**

What creation of the foods you like to eat are you using to validate other people's realities? Everything that is times a godzillion, will you destroy and uncreate it all?

Right and wrong, good and bad, POD and POC, all nine, shorts, boys, and beyonds.

Eating for Comfort

When I invite people to eat only a few bites of their food and stop when their body doesn't want any more, they often realize that from the time they were children, they have eaten for comfort. Eating is the only tactile comfort that many people have. If your family wants to comfort you when you're little, they give you food. They don't ask you what you need, what you want, what you require, or what you desire—they simply give you food.

When babies cry, many parents immediately assume they are hungry and stuff a bottle in their mouth. They don't ask, "Are you hungry?" Even with a little baby, you can ask, "Do you have a dirty diaper? Do you need food? Do you need to be picked up? Do you need to be walked?" and the baby will stop crying when you ask the right question. They know what they need. When my kids were babies, they most often stopped crying when I asked, "Do you need to be walked?" They always wanted to move and never liked staying in one place.

As a child, were you fed when you wanted to be picked up and held or walked around? Were you given food when you were asking for comfort? Does it really comfort you to eat?

Have you misidentified and misapplied that food is for comfort? Everywhere you've bought that food is for comfort when it's really about choice, will you destroy and uncreate all that times a godzillion? Right and wrong, good and bad, POD and POC, all nine, shorts, boys, and beyonds.

When you wanted to be held and rocked to sleep, did you get fed? Once again another form of comfort! Everywhere you have misidentified and misapplied food as comforting energy or as being the same as the comfort you're looking for, will you destroy and uncreate all that times a godzillion? Right and wrong, good and bad, POD and POC, all nine, shorts, boys, and beyonds.

Eating to Cut Off Your Awareness

Many people tell me they overeat to block out their awareness. Someone recently told me, "I became aware that sometimes I eat as a way to manage the psychic input I receive. Eating blocks it out."

How much of your eating are you using to cut off yur awareness? It's just like any other form of addiction. Do you realize you're addicted to eating, and you don't actually need or have a desire to eat? Everything that is times a godzillion, will you destroy and uncreate it all? Right and wrong, good and bad, POD and POC, all nine, shorts, boys, and beyonds.

Tool: Is This Hunger Mine or Someone Else's?

Maybe the feeling you perceive is hunger—but maybe it's not *your* hunger. Maybe it's someone else's. Use this tool: **Is this hunger mine or someone else's?** If it is someone else's, return it to sender and don't eat. Use this tool and save big time on your food bill!

I gave this tool to the people in an obesity class I did awhile ago. A lady who was in the class had been eating donuts at work every day. When she used this tool, she found out she was eating donuts for all the other people in her office who wanted them—not for herself. She stopped eating the donuts that her co-workers wanted—and in one month, she lost twenty pounds.

Tool: Food Cravings

People often ask me about food cravings. Did you know that 90 percent of your food cravings aren't yours? You and your body are aware of other people's energies and desires, which they may have misidentified as well. When you have a food craving, you need to determine:

- *Is this craving what's true for me—or is it what I've bought as true from someone else?*
- *Is it my reality that I crave it? Is it my body's reality? Or is it somebody else's reality that I crave it?*

Everything that is times a godzillion, will you destroy and uncreate it all? Right and wrong, good and bad, POD and POC, all nine, shorts, boys, and beyonds.

Cravings also occur when there's an energy your subtle bodies require. Cravings for food, alcohol, cigarettes, drugs, or anything else stem from an energy the subtle bodies are not getting. The subtle bodies create a physical craving in your body for something that will kick-start and override a barrier to receiving the energy that they want. This may also be true of a craving for sex or other activities. I haven't played with those yet—but it's definitely true of cravings for food.

To overcome the energy block, you can try asking,**"What energies are my subtle bodies not getting that create this craving?"** This may start to change your cravings. You can also POC and POD everything that does not allow your subtle bodies to have the energies they need, require, and desire.

I got over my craving for chocolate by using these tools. I was a total chocoholic. I wanted chocolate all the time. Every time I craved chocolate, I would run, **"Everything that doesn't allow my subtle bodies to get what they require, POC and POD all that."** As I continued to run the process, the cravings went away more and more rapidly. Within about two months, I no longer craved chocolate, and today I eat chocolate occasionally, but the demand that I felt to eat it every day is gone. I used to choose chocolate above anything else—all the time. Now I don't.

Your body knows what it requires and desires. Ask it!

Chapter 8

Positional HEPADs

When you look at your body, how many fixed points of view do you have about it?

Not long ago, Dain worked with a couple that was constantly complaining about each other. He tried all sorts of approaches to help them, but nothing seemed to work. They wouldn't let go of their complaints about each other.

> He said to me, "I can't get anything to change with them. I don't know what's going on."
>
> I said, "You believe they want to change. In reality, they don't want to change anything about themselves. They just want the other person to change."

This often happens. People don't want to change. They want the other person to change so it's right for them. This is what we do with our body as well. Are you expecting your body to change—but you're not willing to change *you*? Do you realize that changing you is what would change your body? Oops!

> A woman said to me, "I feel like I'm fighting a battle with my body. My life and my being are changing, and I'm stepping into a new place and it's 'Body, come along with me! This is fun.' It comes along and everything is good for a while and then it sucker punches me."
>
> I asked, "What are you not being for your body that your body needs you to be that would manifest as the perfect relationship with your body? You have to ask your body to go along with the change you're making, and you also have to look at where you're not willing to change. When you look at where you're not willing to change, you may see how you have created whatever you are resisting."

Any point of view you take about anything creates a position or an outlook in your life—then, without your awareness that position begins to control your life. For example, when you take the position, "This is the perfect man for me," can you see his faults? No, because he's perfect. If you find the "perfect woman," can you see her faults? Nope, she's perfect. When your body seems to be in a battle with you, there are points of view you're not willing to change. We call these positional HEPADs. Positional HEPADs are judgments, conclusions, decisions, points of view, and positions you have taken on. Whenever you say, "I believe *x, y, z.*" you're taking on a positional HEPAD. These are the things we pull together in order to create the limitations in our lives and our body.

HEPADs stands for the handicaps, the entropy, the paralysis, the atrophy, and the destruction that you adopt as a point of view.

- **H**andicaps are things that hamper you. They're disadvantages, deficiencies, or hindrances.

- **E**ntropy is where you take something that has order and ease in it and make it into disorder—something that's chaotic, not comfortable, and not fun.

- **P**aralysis is where you eliminate your choice today in favor of the choice you made yesterday. Have you ever taken the point of view that you couldn't do something? Have you ever said something such as, "I've tried to fix everything in my body and it won't be fixed?" That's paralysis.

- **A**trophy is where you let everything disintegrate because you can't seem to create or control it. Atrophy is what you have to do in order to get old enough to look sick and ugly. You have to atrophy your body—then you begin to destroy it.

- **D**estruction is the way you live your life! You don't get up in the morning and ask, "How can I create me and my body today?" You ask, "What bad thing do I have to take care of today?" You go to the mirror and say, "How awful do I look? Look at the bags under my eyes, look at my sagging chest, look at my sagging butt. How the hell do I get out of here?" This is our form of destruction.

We have positional HEPADs about money, sex, relationships, business—everything—including our bodies. What do the HEPADs do? They create limitations. They don't allow your body to change. Whenever you get vested in a point of view, you're creating HEPADs around how your point of view is right.

Then you make a decision that that's the way things have to be. Once you make a decision, judgment, computation, or conclusion, nothing can come into your awareness that doesn't match it. That's the difficulty with having a point of view.

Your Point of View Does Not Equal You

You may think your points of view equal who you are. This is what most people believe—but it's not true. Your point of view means the finite, limited you. Every point of view you take on limits you. You can take a point of view the way you take a number when you're waiting in line. Here, take a point of view. Take two. They're free. You can take on as many points of view as you wish—or you can have none. Which one feels better to you? None! How can you be what you truly be with no point of view? Well, that's what you truly be—no point of view. When you're being you, you have no point of view. You are being the energy, space, and consciousness that you, as an infinite being, naturally are. If you never take a point of view, what do you have available? Everything! Infinite choice occurs when you have no point of view.

How many positional HEPADs do you have that define everything that is creating your life exactly as it is without the ability to change it? Everything that is, times a godzillion, I destroy and uncreate it all. Right and wrong, good and bad, POD and POC, all nine, shorts, boys, and beyonds.

Clearing HEPADs

Running (or clearing) positional HEPADs is a way to help get your body back to feeling good about itself—and you feeling good about it. It works with pain of any sort- mental, physical, or emotional. Recently I was out riding, and my horse made an unexpected move, which did something strange to my arm. I was in pain for several months, and I kept trying to get rid of it. I had Rolfing, chiropractic, cranial sacral work, and several other things done, but none of it helped. Finally I started to run, "What positional HEPADs am I using to hold this in place?" And it began to unlock. All of a sudden, I remembered falling off a ladder thirty years earlier. I landed on my elbow, cracked it, and dislocated my shoulder all at the same time. I didn't go to the doctor at that time, because I couldn't afford it. Instead I learned to bypass the normal muscle structure so I could use the arm. All of this has been unlocking since I began to run positional HEPADs, and the original muscles are NOW going back into use.

When you are walking and your hip hurts or your leg hurts or your knee or your elbow hurts, instead of saying, "Oh! I've got pain" and trying to recover from it by limping or carrying a cane or walking on crutches, ask, **"How many positional HEPADs do I have holding this in existence?"** Then use the clearing statement.

> *Everything that is times a godzillion, will you destroy and uncreate it all? Right and wrong, good and bad, POD and POC, all nine, shorts, boys, and beyonds.*

"It Breaks My Heart"

You can also run HEPADs on emotional pain. Recently a lady came to do some work with me.

> She said, "I don't know what's wrong with my life. I have no energy. I don't want to do anything. I feel like I can hardly breathe. My life has lost its joy."
>
> I said, "Your life has not lost anything, but you have."
>
> As we worked together, one of the things that came up is that she responded to the things that happened around her with comments like, "Oh, it breaks my heart that this is happening in the world" or "It's heartbreaking that he did this to me."

> I asked, "Do you realize that with that point of view, you're creating congestive heart disease?"

Is this something you do as well? Do you take the position that the world is heartbreaking?

> *What creation of "this is breaking my heart" as reality are you using to lock into existence the positional HEPADs you are choosing? Everything that is times a godzillion, will you destroy and uncreate it all? Right and wrong, good and bad, POD and POC, all nine, shorts, boys, and beyonds.*

Do you respond to things by saying, "Oh, that's so sad. He loves her, but she doesn't love him. She lost her job. That's so sad."? And then do you wonder why *you're* sad? You're sad because things match your point of view that life is sad. What if you took the viewpoint that life was interesting? There's a man out there who is banging his head against a brick wall. "That's an interesting choice."

> *What creation of "that's so sad" are you using to lock into existence the positional HEPADs you are choosing? Everything that is times a godzillion, will you destroy and uncreate it all? Right and wrong, good and bad, POD and POC, all nine, shorts, boys, and beyonds.*

We mindlessly use statements like this all the time. "It's killing me that ____." I knew someone who kept saying, "It beats the shit out of me," then he got colon cancer. Do you ever hear people say, "I'm starving to death"?

Many years ago there was a point where I was getting sick about every three weeks, and I was tired all the time. One day I had an argument with my wife, and as she left the room I said, "I'm frigging sick and tired of this shit!" I suddenly realized I had been thinking that through for months. I was sick and tired all the time. Duh! Am I a great and glorious creator? Yes! So are you. Are you happy with what you are creating? No? Be aware of what you're saying and what you're thinking, because what you're saying and thinking creates your life the way it is. You might want to get clear about your habitual response to things and all the little phrases you throw around.

Working with HEPADs can have very dynamic results. I worked for about six months with a lady who had been diagnosed with cancer. When I met her, she had cancerous masses in her lungs and was getting ready to begin chemo. We started running a simple process: **"What creation of cancerous reality are you using to lock into existence the positional HEPADs you are choosing?"**

After the second or third chemo session, she got an infection, which often happens with chemo, because the immune system becomes so compromised. They took her into the hospital, did an MRI, and discovered that she no longer had any masses in her lungs or anywhere else in her body.

You create cancer—or anything else—and you can uncreate it. You create what's wrong with your body, and you can uncreate it. It's your choice. This can be difficult for most of us, because when we choose something, we try to make it right. We try to figure out why we created it or how it's the right choice rather than realizing, "Okay, that was a stupid choice. I can choose something else." That's really all it takes.

Believing vs. Being Aware

If you create something as a belief, you lock it into reality instead of allowing it to be malleable and changeable. I encourage you to become more malleable and changeable, because if you're willing to change, then you're willing to alter your reality according to what it can be instead of trying to create it the same way day after day. When you try to keep reality always the same, you create limitations that make everything predictable. Every point of view you take creates a position you hold onto, which locks you out of choice.

If you never take a point of view, what do you have available?
Everything! Infinite choice occurs when you have no point of view.

* * *

Additional Processes You Can Do

How many positional HEPADs do you have to make sure you don't know that you know? Everything that is times a godzillion, will you destroy and uncreate it all? Right and wrong, good and bad, POD and POC, all nine, shorts, boys, and beyonds.

How many positional HEPADs do you have to make sure that you can't perceive what you can perceive? Everything that is times a godzillion, will you destroy and uncreate it all? Right and wrong, good and bad, POD and POC, all nine, shorts, boys, and beyonds.

How many positional HEPADs do you have to make sure you can't receive what you can receive? Everything that is times a godzillion, will you destroy and uncreate it all? Right and wrong, good and bad, POD and POC, all nine, shorts, boys, and beyonds.

How many positional HEPADs do you have to make sure you never have to be what you truly be? Everything that is times a godzillion, will you destroy and uncreate it all? Right and wrong, good and bad, POD and POC, all nine, shorts, boys, and beyonds.

We've been creating HEPADs over millions of years, and they exist on many different levels, so it's often beneficial to repeat processes like these many times. You can put these processes on a loop and play it at night while you're sleeping, because you don't have to pay cognitive attention for them to work dynamically.

Chapter 9

Disease, Pain, and Suffering

A lot of people maintain their pain because it allows them feel like other people.

What if pain wasn't a reality but a choice? Do you really want to have pain?

I was recently out riding my new horse. As we went through a river, he stepped on a rock and slid off of it. I fell off, my body hit the rocks, and I experienced an intense crack in my back. I didn't say, "My back is broken" or "I probably won't be able to walk tomorrow." I didn't assume I was going to be hurt or that something was wrong. Instead I asked a question: "What just happened?" Instead of being sore the next day, I discovered that I no longer needed a chiropractor because I have a horse-o-practor. The crack in my back loosened my hips, and they became more comfortable than they have been in years.

You can create a lot of pain and suffering if you take the position that you have been hurt or that you're going to have trouble with your body. Instead, if you take no point of view about an event like this, you can have a different result. I used this approach when my kids were little and they fell down on the sidewalk. I didn't assume they had hurt themselves. I would walk over and ask, "Did you break the concrete?" They would look at the spot where they fell, say *no*, get up, and happily run off again.

My kids never cried when they fell down. They never had bumps on their heads or bruises on their knees like other kids. That's because I had no point of view about what it meant when they fell down. Other parents would watch their child fall down and say, "Oh my God! Are you okay?" How would these kids respond when their parents asked, "Oh, honey! Are you okay?" They'd say, "No, I'm not okay!" and then they would cry for ten minutes. What does this do? It locks the kid into the idea that pain is something one must suffer. Pain is something that one must experience. Pain is the way everybody experiences things. So, if you fall down, then you must have pain. Not true!

Pain Is a Creation

Pain is not real; it's a creation. You create pain. I know this for a fact. Have you ever done fire walking on hot coals? You know what? It doesn't hurt—if you don't decide it's going to hurt. Does this mean we create all the pain in our bodies and the pain in our lives and the pain in everything we do? Yes, it does. We tend to look through the vibrational virtual realities of this reality so that we can feel that we are alike. We have entrained ourselves to be on the same vibration as everyone else, and pain is an entrainment that allows us to believe that we are like other people. If you have people around you who are in pain, you will vibrate to their pain until you create your own version of it.

Fortunately, working with HEPADs can help. Every time you move and you have a pain or stiffness, ask, "How many HEPADs do I have holding this in existence?" Keep doing it as long as anything is resisting—because every resistance you experience is your creation. It doesn't matter why you created it. All that matters is that you created it.

This idea also applies to emotional pain. "He hurt me!" No! He cheated on you. He didn't hurt you. He hurt himself. No one can make you happy. No one can make you sad. No one can hurt your feelings—except you. Wait! Does this mean you're responsible for everything in your life? What a strange concept! It's not just a concept. It is a reality.

> *What creation of pain as reality—physical, emotional, financial, marital, or any kind at all, are you using to lock into existence the positional HEPADs you are choosing? Everything that is times a godzillion, will you destroy and uncreate it all? Right and wrong, good and bad, POD and POC, all nine, shorts, boys, and beyonds.*

You Are One of a Kind

I talked with a woman who was a former dancer. She had a painful injury to her piriformis muscle, which is in the gluteal region. In an attempt to figure out what was going on with her injury, she studied anatomy ad infinitum and bought all the "answers" from all the medical professionals. Every time I asked her to consider a new possibility, she gave me one of the answers she had collected.

> I finally said to her, "Hold on! You're trying to be logical instead of aware. You're giving me somebody else's answer. You think that's real. What if your answer and your creation are based on something that is not real for anybody else? Are you a clone? Is there another person exactly like you in the world?"
>
> She said, "No."

I said, "Right. You're an individual. You are one-of-a-kind. So why are you buying other people's points of view about what's wrong with your body? You're the only one who has a body like yours, you're the only one who has the points of view you have, and you're the only one who can actually see what's going to work for your body. Yet you're buying other people's points of view in order to try and change you. Is that really going to work?"

The points of view she was expressing were positional HEPADs. Every single one of them. This may be something you are doing as well.

How many positional HEPADs do you have to make sure you continue to buy your point of view (from somebody else) about your body or your condition? Everything that is times a godzillion, will you destroy and uncreate it all? Right and wrong, good and bad, POD and POC, all nine, shorts, boys, and beyonds.

What Has Changed?

The same woman was doing something else that people sometimes do with their injuries or pain. As she delineated every location where the pain "belonged," I could feel her locking it in place. She didn't stop to become aware or to test to see if the pain had changed. Instead she asked, "Do I still have it?" This is not a good approach. Of course you still have it, because you can create anything! "Do I still have it?" is not a question. You're assuming that you still have it—and then you attach a question mark at the end of your assumption.

The thing to do is ask, "What has changed?" "What am I going to be, do, have, create, or generate for this to change?" Not for it to go away—for it to change.

I said to her, "You've got to look. You've got to say, 'Okay, I chose this. I would choose this for what reason? Was this a good choice? I chose to make the right side of my body an atrophied pile of crap so I can prove that I can dance no matter how much pain I'm in. I can overcome all obstacles and still be beautiful, wonderful and fabulous.' Those are all HEPADs you have taken on."

Look at what you have taken on without justifying or explaining anything. You have become very good at locking these things into existence. HEPADs are a creation. You've been creating them for billions or trillions of years. You have to work with them patiently. You can't just demand that they go away.

What creation of the rightness and wrongness—especially of you—as reality are you using to lock into existence the positional HEPADs you are choosing? Everything that is times a godzillion, will you destroy and uncreate it all? Right and wrong, good and bad, POD and POC, all nine, shorts, boys, and beyonds.

Giving Things a Name

We assume that giving a name to our aches, pains, or whatever we have is the correct and usual thing to do. You feel something and you say, "Oh, I have a pain" or "I have a virus" or "I have a pulled muscle." No, that's not what you have. You have an awareness. Instead of giving your awareness a name or looking for a diagnosis, (which is an answer), go into the question. Thank your body for the awareness and ask:

- *Okay, what can I do with this?*
- *Can I change it?*
  If you get a yes to that question, ask: How do I change it?

Then use the tools in your toolbox HEPADs, POC and POD, "Who Does This Belong To?" or whatever is going to work.

I talked with someone who told me she has a problem because of her low self-esteem. I asked, "What question is the statement, 'I have this problem because of my low self-esteem'? That's an answer and your justification for why you have the problem. But you created the problem. You can't change anything you don't have a question about! All you can do is reiterate your answer as though your answer is the truth. If you want to change something, ask a question about it, then change it."

How many positional HEPADs do you have to keep the psychological mumbo jumbo that you use to justify all your limitations in existence? A lot? A little or megatons? Beyond megatons? Everything that is times a godzillion, will you destroy and uncreate it all? Right and wrong, good and bad, POD and POC, all nine, shorts, boys, and beyonds.

Pain Is a Way to Avoid Awareness

Many people use pain, upsets, and tears as a way of avoiding awareness. We choose pain, unhappiness, and tears as a way to not be aware of what we are aware of. We create pain to avoid awareness.

Have you ever gotten spacey when you had pain? You go to a place where what you experience seems like pain then you go beyond it and all of a sudden you feel sort of spacey, dizzy, or out of it. What is that? It's the intensity of space that is available to you, which you try to avoid because you assume that intensity equals pain. It's a beautiful thing to have and be all that space, and that we so assiduously avoid it. It's completely crazy.

- *When you're in pain, try asking:*
- *What awareness am I avoiding with the pain I am choosing?*
- *What awareness am I avoiding with the tears I am using?*
- *What awareness am I avoiding with the unhappiness I am choosing?*

What are you using and perpetrating on your body as an avoidance of awareness? Everything that is times a godzillion, will you destroy and uncreate it all? Right and wrong, good and bad, POD and POC, all nine, shorts, boys, and beyonds.

Have You Tried to Ignore Pain?

Have you tried to walk past pain as though it doesn't exist? Have you tried to overcome your pain by ignoring it? Have you stood 5,000 miles outside your body in order to avoid feeling what your body feels? I've done all those things. They don't work. Ignoring pain is different from saying, "Wow! This is intense." What if you didn't refuse or ignore that sensation but instead enjoyed it and asked:

- *Okay body, what do you need from me here?*
- *What do you require?*
- *What do you desire?*
- *What are you telling me that I'm not willing to hear?*

Do You Hold onto Pain?

Some people hold onto pain. They maintain their pain because it allows them to feel like other people. Or they become so identified with their pain that they don't know who they would be without it. How do you get out of holding onto pain? Ask yourself:

- *Do I really need this pain?*
- *What am I using this pain for?*

Oftentimes when people come out of pain that they've had for a long while, they feel that something is wrong. This happened to me. Years ago I got Rolfed, and one morning after the fifth Rolfing (a specific type of massage) session, I woke up and thought something was wrong. What was "wrong" was I no longer had the pain in my body that had been there for 25 years. Being without it was so unfamiliar to me that something seemed amiss. The wrongness of no pain and the rightness of no change is the way people consistently function on planet Earth. When you are aware, you can get to the point where you're willing to change and live without pain.

We resist other kinds of change as well. Do you ever want the people in your life to stay the same—and not change? Do people ever try to get you to stay in the same position, to have the same point of view or to do the same thing, even though it doesn't work for you any more?

This sort of thing sometimes happens with young people as they grow up. As they begin to go into puberty, they have a reaction like, "Oh no! I'm changing" as though it's wrong. It's the same with aging. There is nothing wrong with any of it. It's a wrongness based in VVRs—not reality.

It's interesting to me that pleasure has such a charge on it. How many people do you see who live pleasurable lives? How many people do you see who live painful lives? Many people seem to think that the pain of life proves they're actually having a life. They don't believe that the pleasure and the joy they take in living is what proves they're having a life.

> *What physical actualization of the terminal, eternal, and infectious disease of the choice of the CCCRs for the creation of the wrongness of no pain and the rightness of no change do you have that maintains and entrains everything that you cannot change, choose, and institute as the total joy in living? Everything that is times a godzillion, will you destroy and uncreate it all? Right and wrong, good and bad, POD and POC, all nine, shorts, boys, and beyonds.*

Your Body Is a Sensory Organ

A woman told me that she had been traveling for her work and she began to have symptoms of nephritis, which is an inflammation of the kidneys. It was the first time she had any issues with her kidneys.

> I asked, "Who did you come into contact with who had that?"

She was not aware of being in contact with anyone who had nephritis.

> I said, "The problem is that you are way more aware than you give yourself credit for."

When you come across people who have something wrong with their bodies, your body is aware of it. If you ignore that, you can lock what is wrong with *their* body into *your* body. Your body is saying, "Listen to me, I'm telling you what's wrong with this person!" If you make the mistake of saying, "Oh no, I like this person. There's nothing wrong with him or her," your body's going to say, "You need to know this person has a problem." Your body is a sensory organ. It is designed to give you information. We don't use it that way. We abuse it by ignoring it.

> When I'm around somebody who I know has a pain in their body, I say, "Can I just hold my hand on your back for a minute?"
>
> They'll ask, "Why?"
>
> I'll say, "Well, don't you have some pain there?"
>
> They'll ask, "How did you know that?" which is pretty funny, because their body is yelling at me, "Help, help! I have pain! Fix me! You can fix me."

Do I want to have a strange body screaming at me all the time? No, so I'll just put my hand where they have the pain or I'll ask, "Can I give you a hug?"

Running HEPADs on Other People

Someone asked me if it is appropriate to run HEPADs on spouses and children. I said, "Do anything that makes your life better. Will it work? Maybe. But remember that they are as stubborn as you are. That's why they're your children and your spouse."

Someone else asked, "Can HEPADs be run at a distance?" The answer is yes; however, you can't do anything for or to people that they're not willing to receive. You can work your arse off, and if they don't truly want it, it ain't going to work. If they *do* want it, it will work. If you're doing it because you want to fix them, give it up. It's not going to happen. You can't fix anyone.

When you try to help someone, you are always coming from a position of superiority. Help requires you to judge someone as less than you. Sympathy, empathy and compassion all require you to judge the same way. People choose what they choose. Why they choose it, you won't know. Is it wrong or sad that they choose it? No, it's just what they choose. If someone doesn't ask for help, don't try to help.

A while ago, I saw a little old lady who had been standing on a street corner for a long time. I decided to help her cross the street, because I decided she obviously needed help. I walked over to her and asked, "Can I help you cross the street?"

> She said, "I don't need your help," and she hit me with her cane.
>
> I said, "Okay, I was just doing superiority. Excuse me. I'm sorry."

She didn't need help. She wasn't asking for help—and if somebody's not asking, don't offer. But—this doesn't mean that they don't ask silently. Some of them do. So you have to be aware.

Everything you've done and everything you've created to try to fix another as though that's going to make everything all right, times a godzillion, will you destroy and uncreate it all? Right and wrong, good and bad, POD and POC, all nine, shorts, boys, and beyonds.

Duplicating Your Parent's Symptoms

I talked with a woman who told me she was having problems with the nerve endings in her hands and feet. She said she was having pain and was unable to firmly grip things.

> I asked her, "So how much of that is actually yours, and how much of it belongs to some old lady that you're trying to take care of?"

She realized that almost none of it belonged to her. She was trying to take care of her mother. It is not uncommon for people to decide that they are their mother or their father and to take their parent's symptoms into their body. It's a psychological symptom that becomes a physical symptom when they take it on.

I worked with another lady in Texas who was taking her mother's symptoms into her body. As we worked together, she recognized what she was doing, but we couldn't get her to fully let go of the symptoms. We had to find a way to deal with what her body was choosing, which was to take care of her mother by adopting her symptoms.

You might have a parent whose body you took on. Or you might have taken on the beingness of a parent you didn't want to be like. You decided you had to duplicate them in order to determine how *not* to be like them, but in the process of duplicating them, you became them, and locked all of that into your body.

> *How many of the problems you're having with your body are because you've duplicated one of your parents in order to not be like them? Everything that is times a godzillion, will you destroy and uncreate it all? Right and wrong, good and bad, POD and POC, all nine, shorts, boys, and beyonds.*

The Ambiguity Process

When you're dealing with pain, illness, and suffering, being ambiguous becomes important. Ask questions about what's going on with your body. Avoid decisions and conclusions, like the woman who concluded she was having nerve problems. Use the ambiguity process and ask:

- *What is this?*
- *What can I do with it?*
- *Can I change it?*
- *How do my body and I change it?*

I'm inviting you to be in communion with your body. Being ambiguous—asking questions—is the way to do that.

Universal Surrogate

Universal surrogate is a job title many people take on. A universal surrogate is someone who swears for the rest of his or her life, for all eternity, he or she will take on the pain and suffering of others in order to make everybody well and happy. It's like a blood oath. You vow to take on other people's cancer, pain, suffering, disease, weight, unhappiness, and misery so they can be happy. You become a high priest or priestess as the universal surrogate.

Would you like to give up all the oaths, vows, swearings, fealties, comealties[ix]*, and commitments? Everything that is times a godzillion, will you destroy and uncreate it all? Right and wrong, good and bad, POD and POC, all nine, shorts, boys, and beyonds.*

Once when I was doing an animal class, I worked with a woman who had a dog that kept getting cancer. She would take it to the vet and cut out the cancer, and the dog would get cancer again.

ix See the Glossary for definitions of *fealities* and *comealties*.

> I realized the dog was a surrogate and I asked, "Who is the dog taking the cancer out of?"
>
> I said, "Dog, will you please stop doing that. They won't be able to cure the person if you keep taking the cancer out of them."
>
> The dog said, "Oh, okay," and it quit.

Two weeks later they found out that the grandmother had stage four bone cancer. She died shortly after that. Had she known earlier she might have been able to do something about it, but because she was able to give it to her dog—and the dog was willing to receive it—she didn't hurt, and she didn't feel bad. The dog was removing the pain and suffering of the cancer from her body, but the cancer was still there. It was growing dynamically—she just wasn't feeling it.

If you take on other people's pain and suffering-psychologically, mentally, physically, emotionally, whatever way you do it—you're crippling them and preventing them from changing.

Tool: Return to Sender:

Don't take other people's suffering into your body. When you perceive other people's pain, suffering, emotions, and judgments, return them to sender. You return them to sender to stop the flow of that kind of energy towards you. If you don't return it, they'll keep sending it to you, and they'll never get rid of it or get over it themselves. When you return the lies or the disease (or whatever it is) to sender, you're inviting them to have the awareness that the pain and suffering is there so they can choose something different—if they wish to.

Donnielle told me about a time she was in JFK airport. Her heart started to hurt, and she thought, "Oh my gosh! My heart is hurting." In that split second, she could see a future of doctor's visits, shortness of breath, difficulty walking, surgeries, and all that. Then she said, "Wait a minute. I don't have heart problems. Who does this belong to?" She returned the heart problems to sender with consciousness attached. (You don't have to know where something comes from to do this. Sometimes you may figure out where it comes from, sometimes you don't.) Right after this, Donnielle noticed that there was an elderly couple a short distance away. The woman turned to husband and asked, "Honey, is your heart hurting?"

She saw that her body was trying to help the man, and she almost bought his problem as her own. She said, "I could have created a future of heart problems for myself, but I went, 'Wait a minute! That's not mine!'"

You're far more psychic than you realize, which is a good thing, but because you're not taught to value how aware you are or what to do with your awareness, you might believe that this kind of awareness is a bad thing. It's not a bad thing! The problem occurs when you misidentify other people's pain, suffering, disease, phobias, emotions, and judgments as yours when they aren't! Just return them to sender.

You're an individual. You are one-of-a-kind.
So why are you buying other people's points of view
about what's wrong with your body?

* * *

Additional Tools and Processes You Can Use

Disease

Do you believe in disease? How cool is that? You get to be sick and go to the doctor so he can tell you what to do, how to do it, and when to do it.

What creation of disease as reality are you using to lock into existence the positional HEPADs you are choosing? Everything that is times a godzillion, will you destroy and uncreate it all? Right and wrong, good and bad, POD and POC, all nine, shorts, boys, and beyonds.

Tool: What Are You Sick Of?

My son was getting sick all the time and I asked him, "What are you sick of?"

He said, "I'm sick of this, this, and this."

"Okay," I thought to myself, "Destroy and uncreate that." I didn't say it out loud because he doesn't like Access Consciousness. I asked him again, "So, what else are you sick of?

He answered, and I said, "Okay. What else are you sick of? Cool. Can you let go of that?"

He said, "Sure."

We continued until he had no more answers. The next day I called him and asked, "How you feeling today?"

He said, "I'm well now."

I asked, "Do you think it has anything to do with what we did yesterday?"

He said, "What did we do yesterday?"

It had no relationship to him.

Where are you assuming that whatever you are sick of has nothing to do with what's creating your life the way it is?

What are you sick of about your body? Everything that is times a godzillion, will you destroy and uncreate it all? Right and wrong, good and bad, POD and POC, all nine, shorts, boys, and beyonds.

Are you sick of being old? Are you sick of being tired? Sick of being sick? Sick of being pressured? Sick of people telling you what to do about your weight, what to do about your body, or how to live your life? Are you sick of being told you're wrong? Everything that is times a godzillion, will you destroy and uncreate it all? Right and wrong, good and bad, POD and POC, all nine, shorts, boys, and beyonds.

Chapter 10

Olding And Aging

It takes a tremendous amount of energy to make your body as old as you've decided it is.

You age your body according to the chronological age your body becomes. When you're ten years old, it's "Oh! Now I have two numbers in my age." When you turn thirteen, it's "I'm a teenager now." When you're eighteen, you're one thing—and then you're nineteen and you're something else. As you get closer to new ages, you put points of view in place about what it means to have your body be that age. You have points of view about what you're supposed to look like when you're x number of years old. Some of these viewpoints were created when you were a kid. When you turned eighteen, you might have said, "I'm getting old" because, depending on where you lived, you were then able to vote or buy liquor. Or maybe you decided you were getting old when you turned thirty or forty.

Birthdays

Aging and olding is something that we celebrate from the time we're little. It's called a birthday. You celebrate every year that passes, and then eventually you get old and die. You do not celebrate generative embodiment, which is where you're living each day from the joy of it. You have the joy of your body in each and every moment. This is very different from focusing on having a life or completing a stage of life.

Do you realize that every time you celebrate your birthday (becoming a year older), you're creating a system that causes you to create the life span you currently have and to function in ways that do not give you generative life? You celebrate destruction of your body because you age it and old it each time you celebrate a birthday. This is the problem with celebrating birthdays. If you like to celebrate, celebrate generative embodiment every year instead of your birthday and see what kind of things result.

> *What physical actualization of the terminal, eternal, and infectious disease of the celebration of olding and aging do you have that maintains and entrains what you cannot change, choose, and institute as totally generative embodiment? Everything that is times a godzillion, will you destroy and uncreate it all? Right and wrong, good and bad, POD and POC, all nine, shorts, boys, and beyonds.*

Vibrational Virtual Realities and Aging

Most of us look at the configuration of our body based on the vibrational virtual realities of this reality, which tell us what's supposed to happen when we get to a certain age. They're standards for what's supposed to happen as we age. For example, your hormones are supposed to diminish, which means menopause, stress fractures, osteoporosis, and all those things that are supposed to happen. We say, "I'm forty years old so I will lose my eyesight. I'm fifty years old so will lose estrogen. I'm seventy years old so I will lose testosterone." This is the result that makes you think you don't care about sex any more after you go through menopause or man-o-pause, and think you have lost your desire for sex. This occurs on both sides of the game, both male and female.

It's also what impels puberty, and it's probably what makes men grow hair out of their ears, out of their arse, and out of their nose as they age. Hormonal balances may also pertain to why we have trouble losing weight or generating our bodies to become a different shape. We supposedly stop creating growth hormones, which create muscular, toned bodies. The thing is, your hormonal balances change according to your point of view. If you change your point of view, you change your hormones. Many people have told me they lost weight after they changed their points of view, which undoubtedly changed the balance of hormones in their body and created a different reality. In other words, when we buy into the points of view that everyone has about aging, we create the hormonal standards for our body.

A number of years ago, my joints were getting stiff and my knees hurt every time I walked up and down stairs. I went to a wellness center where they did some blood tests.

> The doctor said, "Your growth hormone level is that of an eighty-five-year-old man."
>
> I asked, "So, what do I do?"
>
> He said, "You need to take injections of human growth hormone."
>
> I said, "Okay."
>
> He said, "Once you start, you'll have to take them forever."
>
> I asked, "Really? I have to take them forever?"
>
> He said, "Yes, once you start them, you have to keep them up."

I injected human growth hormone into my thigh for about three months, and at the beginning of the fourth month, I went to stab myself in the leg, and my body jerked away so hard, I couldn't get the needle in. No matter what I did, I could not get my leg to stand still long enough to get the needle in.

> I asked my body, "What's the matter? Don't you want this?"
>
> It said, "No!"
>
> I asked, "Okay, can you create your own growth hormones?"
>
> It said, "Yes."
>
> I said, "What? The doctor said that's not possible."
>
> My body said, "I ain't taking those shots."

So I stopped taking the growth hormone. That was several years ago, and I haven't had any problems with my knees since then. My body is apparently now creating its own growth hormones.

What physical actualization of the terminal and eternal disease of the creation of hormonal standards solely and only through the VVRs of this reality do you have that maintains and entrains what you cannot change, choose, and institute as the hormonal balance, generation, and creation your body requires and desires? Everything that is times a godzillion, will you destroy and uncreate it all? Right and wrong, good and bad, POD and POC, all nine, shorts, boys, and beyonds.

All the points of view that you have created or generated or have locked into your body that keep you from having a hormonal balance that is the correct generation and creation for your body, will you now destroy and uncreate all those? Right and wrong, good and bad, POD and POC, all nine, shorts, boys, and beyonds.

Dying in the Beauty of Youth

There are people who dread the idea of aging and decide that they don't want to live beyond a certain age. There was a society of people that included the English poets Keats, Shelley, and Byron, who wanted to die in the beauty of their youth. Do you want to die while you are still young and beautiful like Marilyn Monroe? Do you not want to die old and ugly? You might want to check with people who are doing the dying in the beauty of youth thing and ask:

What physical actualization of the terminal and eternal disease of dying while beautiful and having a beautiful death do you have that maintains and entrains what you cannot change, choose, and institute as total generative embodiment and indefinite life? Everything that is times a godzillion, will you destroy and uncreate it all? Right and wrong, good and bad, POD and POC, all nine, shorts, boys, and beyonds.

Drop Dead by (Date)

Have you locked in a drop dead by (date)? Have you had your drop dead by (date) imprinted on your soul? On your body? In your reality? In your psyche?

On my mother's eightieth birthday, she told me, "No one should live to be older than eighty-one" It was a decision she had made. Her father died when he was eighty-one, after his kids decided it was time for him to retire. Without his permission or agreement, they took away his team of horses and sold them. He had loved driving his horses and plowing his fields. The old man was tough as nails and probably would have lived to be one hundred years old, but the loss of his horses killed him.

> When my mother told me this, I asked, "Does this mean you're going to die next year, mom?"
>
> She said, "Nope, I'm just telling you no one should live to be older than eighty-one."

I started visiting her more often, knowing that she had just given me her drop-dead by date. When she was eighty and a half years old, she went in for an operation. They gave her anesthesia—and her mind went away. She was gone. I later found out that her doctor had her on Valium for 38 years—a little long to be doing that—and the anesthesia put her over the edge. She was not competent after that. We put her into a rest home, and she started to die. About a month after her eighty-first birthday, she was dead. She had been totally healthy. She had great verve and vitality. At eighty, she could run up and down stairs—she could outwalk me. But she had decided she was supposed to die when she was eighty-one—so she did.

Living Indefinitely

In this reality, the idea is that you get older and wiser. Is that true? Do you get older and wiser? Or do you get more weary, tired, and jaded? You get older, more world-weary, and dedicated to societal structures. Societal structures are about ensuring you don't have the sense that there is a different choice. You go towards where everybody else is going. Becoming dedicated to societal norms is to kill your body—not to generate it. It's to get old—not to have an indefinite life.

Indefinite living is different from eternal life. It is living totally until you decide you don't want to live any more. It's a different reality from, "I don't want to die." It means you get to choose when you die. You don't have to be immortal. You don't have to live forever. You just get to choose and say, "Okay, you know what? Enough."

Until that time comes, I'm living indefinitely. I get up every day and it's a question: "What do I get to do today?" It's not: "What do I have to do today?" I don't do things I don't want to do. Does this mean that those things don't get done? No. I ask somebody else to do them!

Years ago when I was in the upholstery business, I went to the house of a lady who was redecorating. She said, "I'm ninety-two years old, and I may not live to see the end of this project—but I'm redecorating my house." She got up every morning at six o'clock, she read until eight then she went out and worked with the gardener in her garden. She was vibrant and active. She was still driving and doing all the things that people ten years younger had stopped doing.

When I was in the horse business in my twenties, I met a ninety-year-old man who went out every day to ride his five-year-old saddlebred gelding. The horse was so tall—and the man was so small—that he had to stand on a four-foot tack box in order to get on the horse. He'd mount the horse and go racing up and down the avenue. I always thought he was going to fall off, but he never did.

I said, "That's where I want to be when I'm ninety years old. I want to be getting on a horse and riding, regardless." Those kinds of decisions create a life where you are generative. You're living indefinitely. You're not looking at how you are getting old.

What physical actualization of the terminal and eternal disease of the choice for the CCCRs for the creation of societal structures in existence that destroys bodies and doesn't generate them do you have that maintains and entrains what you cannot change, choose, and institute as a radically different physical embodiment? Everything that is times a godzillion, will you destroy and uncreate it all? Right and wrong, good and bad, POD and POC, all nine, shorts, boys, and beyonds.

Youthenizing

Right now we function from the point of view that we get older year by year. What if that were not true? What if you didn't have to be your "so-called" age? What if you were old enough to have indefinite life—not in the configuration of this reality? What if a "year" was not an appropriate form of measurement? What if we got younger year by year? Totally radical, generative embodiment might be able to reverse the flow of aging. You may want to consider that as a possibility.

What physical actualization of the terminal and eternal disease of the creation of olding and aging of bodies solely and only through the vibrational virtual realities of this reality do you have that maintains and entrains what you cannot change, choose, and institute as a totally generative body, a totally youthenizing body, and indefinite living? Everything that is times a godzillion, will you destroy and uncreate it all? Right and wrong, good and bad, POD and POC, all nine, shorts, boys, and beyonds.

What creation of bodies as olding, aging, decaying, and degenerating as reality are you using to lock into existence the positional HEPADs you are choosing to not have indefinite life? Everything that is times a godzillion, will you destroy and uncreate it all? Right and wrong, good and bad, POD and POC, all nine, shorts, boys, and beyonds.

A Wise Woman

Years ago, I was in Hollywood and I saw the actress Mae West. She was well into her eighties, and she had had so many facelifts that she didn't have a wrinkle—but she had lost all the mobility in her face. She couldn't smile. All she could do was open her mouth to talk and blink her eyes, which were heavily made up with false eyelashes. She was corseted and wearing a gown and a fur coat. She looked like a wax figure from Madame Tussauds. Why do people think that's attractive? It's as if they're trying to stick themselves in one moment in time. And if you choose to stick yourself in one moment in time, where would you be living? Would you be living *then*—or would you be living *now*? My point of view is that you'd better be living now.

A wise woman is a woman who has no point of view about how she looks. She is ageless and timeless. She can dress sexy and look good and do all the right things, and she doesn't care about it. Will she take care of her hair and maybe dye it? She might. Will she present herself in outrageous outfits? Sometimes. Will she do whatever is necessary? Yes—because she is a leader in the movement of women instead of being a follower. If you try to make yourself into the Joan Rivers version of a woman, then you are a follower. You try to look like you're thirty-five forever. Why would you want to do that? The same is true for wise men.

* * *

Additional Processes You Can Do

What physical actualization of the terminal and eternal disease of the creation of bodies between eighteen and eighty do you have that maintains and entrains what you cannot change, choose, and institute as the creation of your body? Everything that is times a godzillion, will you destroy and uncreate it all? Right and wrong, good and bad, POD and POC, all nine, shorts, boys, and beyonds.

What physical actualization of the terminal and eternal disease of the creation of body configuration solely and only through the vibrational virtual realities of this reality do you have that maintains and entrains what you cannot change, choose, and institute as a totally different configuration of your body? Everything that is times a godzillion, will you destroy and uncreate it all? Right and wrong, good and bad, POD and POC, all nine, shorts, boys, and beyonds.

What physical actualization of the terminal and eternal disease of the choice of the CCCRs for the creation of the line-age and the signage on your face do you have that maintains and entrains everything you cannot change, choose, and institute as a totally smooth and youthenizing visage? Everything that is times a godzillion, will you destroy and uncreate it all? Right and wrong, good and bad, POD and POC, all nine, shorts, boys, and beyonds.

What creation of bad eyesight as reality are you using to lock into existence the positional HEPADs you are choosing about what you're not willing to perceive, know, be, and receive? Everything that is times a godzillion, will you destroy and uncreate it all? Right and wrong, good and bad, POD and POC, all nine, shorts, boys, and beyonds.

What creation of diminished capacity for hearing as reality are you using to lock into existence the positional HEPADs you are choosing to not perceive, know, be, and receive? Everything that is times a godzillion, will you destroy and uncreate it all? Right and wrong, good and bad, POD and POC, all nine, shorts, boys, and beyonds.

Here's another one for those of you like me, who are getting older. You can use this as Access Botox.

What physical actualization of the terminal and eternal disease of the choice of the CCCRs for the creation of stresses for defining the lines on your face do you have that maintains and entrains the proof of the wisdom of life? Everything that is times a godzillion, will you destroy and uncreate it all? Right and wrong, good and bad, POD and POC, all nine, shorts, boys, and beyonds.

I started running the process below on myself and all of a sudden, I had more energy. My tendons didn't hurt as much, and I didn't feel quite so old. Try it and see what happens for you.

What creation of bodies as olding, aging, degenerating, and decaying as reality are you using to lock into existence the positional HEPADs you are choosing for death? Everything that is times a godzillion, will you destroy and uncreate it all? Right and wrong, good and bad, POD and POC, all nine, shorts, boys, and beyonds.

Chapter 11

Owning Your Money, Your Body, And Your Life

Everything about money is about taking care of your body.
And everything about your body is about taking care of your money.

I had often thought that there was a correlation between money and the body, but I had not realized the correlation between them was so deep until a friend and I were looking at the way she never owned her money. She had the point of view that if she was taking money for the work she did, she was taking something she shouldn't have. This is insane, but we have more insane points of view than we have sane points of view (in case you haven't noticed). We ran a process about this, and about a week later, she said, "I don't understand it. My body lost four pounds in the last week."

She had another very interesting result. She had always been untidy. Her space was total disorder; her things were strewn around and everything was in disarray. After we ran this process, she started to put things away. She began to hang up her clothes. Everything was neatly folded.

> She said, "The chaos I used to create in my life is not there any more. Now I like everything to be neat, tidy, and orderly."
>
> I said, "That's because you now own your money, your body, your possessions, and your space. Everything about money is about taking care of your body—and everything about your body is about taking care of your money."

If you don't own your own money, you can't own your own body. You need money to handle your clothing, your food and, your car. All of those things are related to your body. They're not related to you, the being. And they all require money. Money is about taking care of your body; it's not about anything else. Ninety-nine percent of the things you do with money have to do with taking care of your body.

When you don't have a sense that you own your money, you don't trust yourself to generate it. It's also likely that you don't own your body. You may not even know what it means to own your body. When you were a kid, were you given money—but not allowed to spend it the way you wanted to? Were you told to be in control of your body—but made to go to bed when you didn't wish to? Were you made to eat what you didn't like? This takes away your sense of empowerment with your body. You don't see that you have choice with your body or real control of it. You may not even have a true desire for those things. All of this is about not owning your body.

Do you have the point of view that you don't like a certain part of your body? That's an indication that you don't own your body. Ask, **"What part of my body do I own?"** Many people who are very intellectual have the point of view that the only part of their body they own is their head. That's the part they think they control. If they grew up in a family where they weren't allowed to control their body, they discovered they could always control things in their head. They would focus on what they could think about—what they could do with their head—that no one else could see or catch. These are the ways we begin to abdicate ownership of our body.

When my kids were young, I let them be in control of their bodies as much as possible. Once when my youngest son was two years old, I told him it was time for bed.

> He said, "No bed! Watch television!"
>
> I said, "It's really time for you to go to bed. Are you ready to go to bed?"
>
> He said, "No!"
>
> I said, "Well, okay, I'm going to bed. I'll see you in the morning. Turn off the lights when you are finished."

About half an hour later, he turned off the lights and put himself to bed. It was the last time he ever fought me about going to bed because he realized he was on his own, and he didn't like it that much. Today he's someone who owns his body.

Some people don't have ownership of their body around food. Many of us were made to eat everything on our plates. When someone else imposes on you what you have to eat, you give up ownership of your body. By the time the youngest of my four kids came along, I was too tired to worry about what she ate. I'd say, "Just go to the refrigerator and get whatever you want." She was drinking Cokes when she was three years old, but very shortly after that, when she could have anything she wanted, she started eating vegetables. She now eats better than all my other kids because the other kids fought against the "healthy food" I tried to impose on them—and she was allowed to eat whatever her body desired. She grazed all day long. Kids will graze all day long—if you let them. Were you allowed to graze as a kid? Or did you have to sit down to meals and eat four squares a day?

> *What energy, space, and consciousness can you and your body be for you to own your money with total ease? Everything that doesn't allow that to show up times a godzillion, will you destroy and uncreate it all? Right and wrong, good and bad, POD and POC, all nine, shorts, boys, and beyonds.*

> *What physical actualization of the terminal and eternal disease of the choice of the CCCRs for the creation of never owning your own money or your own body do you have that maintains and entrains what you cannot be, do, have, create, generate, change, choose, and institute as the reality of your body? Everything that is times a godzillion, will you destroy and uncreate it all? Right and wrong, good and bad, POD and POC, all nine, shorts, boys, and beyonds.*

Repetitive Patterns

Years ago, I looked at my life, and realized that I kept doing the same things over and over again. I could see the repetitive patterns I kept carrying out. I started asking, "How the heck did I get to the place where everything stays the same instead of becoming what it could be?" We all have repetitive patterns in our lives. We also have repetitive patterns with our bodies. We go onto automatic pilot and create our body from repetitive patterns, as though that creates possibility—but it doesn't. We do repetitive patterns rather than choosing to change. We use our patterns as a checkout point from awareness. These patterns are based on the supposedly correct purposes and systems that society has established on planet Earth. When you lock into repetitive patterns, you are not owning your body, your money, or your life.

Recently I talked with a woman about repetitive patterns and she said, "What's coming up for me as a repetitive pattern is marriage." Now there's a repetitive pattern! There are even oaths and vows in the marriage ceremony that you agree to keep in place until death do you part. It may be that in many different lifetimes, including this one, you've given over control of your body and your money to someone else, either through marriage, friendship, relationship, sex, or copulation. There are a thousand ways in which we do this.

The traditional secret agenda of marriage is that if you're a woman and you have property, you give it to your man. If your man has property, he gives up nothing to you. You, as a woman, are a valueless product unless you have children. Would that be owning your own body or not owning your own body? If you haven't had children, you're not owning your body—and if you have had children, you're not owning your body—because your kids own it now. That's a real win-win situation, isn't it? Children then expect you to take care of them. They expect you to take care of all of their physical problems and all of their difficulties, which means you get to own their bodies. And they get to own your body or to have control over your money and your body. In the end, no one wins.

If you're a woman and have spent the last 10,000 years getting married and giving up your property as a repetitive pattern, it's likely that you may do that again this lifetime, because that's the way it's done. It's as though it's a given—but nothing has to be a given. Everything should be malleable, mutable, and changeable. Unfortunately, that's not the way most of us function. I know too many women who have given up their lives for their families and their husbands. Then they get resentful. They get divorced and they hate their ex-husband—but he wasn't the one who made them give up their life. They chose to give it up.

I've noticed that in some families the cycle of abuse is consistent and repetitive. People have a willingness to be abused in every relationship they are involved in. They go through one relationship after another—and all of them are abusive. They keep choosing that, because that's the cycle they've seen and the cycle they've lived—and that's the cycle they function from. It's a repetitive pattern.

Most people take on a relationship that is like the relationship they had in the beginning of their lives, whether it's abusive or constructive. When you do that, you're not owning your body. You're not creating or choosing your body—or your life.

What physical actualization of the terminal, eternal, and infectious disease of the choice of the CCCRs for the creation of consistent repetitive patterns for the creation of bodies and life do you have that maintains and entrains what you absolutely cannot be, do, have, create, generate, change, choose, and institute as a totally different possibility, choice, and life? Everything that is times a godzillion, will you destroy and uncreate it all? Right and wrong, good and bad, POD and POC, all nine, shorts, boys, and beyonds.

How much of what you do with your body is a repetitive pattern? All the repetitive patterns you've done in every frigging lifetime to create bodies, will you destroy and uncreate all that? Right and wrong, good and bad, POD and POC, all nine, shorts, boys, and beyonds.

Inherited Money

Have you observed people who inherit money? Have you noticed that they often quickly find ways to get rid of it? They invest it badly, give it away, or find some way of losing it. Never owning your own money is one of the reasons why, when you inherit money, you get rid of it. You have decided you can't own something you didn't create. You don't own the inherited money, and you don't own your body either, because your parents are responsible for the creation of it. This is another repetitive pattern from generation to generation, lifetime to lifetime.

Would an infinite being choose to do the same thing more than once? Probably not, but we keep doing repetitive patterns as though we're going to get well, get better, or get something. I just don't know what the *something* is. Living is not about going with the pattern. It's about going with the flow of energy.

> *What energy, space, and consciousness can you and your body be that would allow you to be the joyful, expansive energy you truly be? Everything that is times a godzillion, will you destroy and uncreate it all? Right and wrong, good and bad, POD and POC, all nine, shorts, boys, and beyonds.*

You Have to Be the Energy of Everything

The idea is that in order to *have* anything you have to be willing to *be* anything. You have to be the energy of everything. When you buy the idea that you don't own your own money or you don't own your own body, you essentially deny everything you truly are as an infinite being. Instead of being you, you create repetitive patterns as if that is who you are.

What repetitive patterns do your body and you have that keep you in existence? Everything that is times a godzillion, will you destroy and uncreate it all? Right and wrong, good and bad, POD and POC, all nine, shorts, boys, and beyonds.

The Pattern of Saying No as a First Response

When you were a kid, you may have learned that the only time you could manage to have any sense of owning your life or your body or your money was when you said *no.* You learned that being negative was the way to have a sense of you. That became a repetitive pattern. This would explain why people consistently choose to make themselves wrong. They look at the negative of themselves instead of seeing that they have value. They look at the wrongness, because that's the way they create a sense of their own reality.

How many repetitive patterns do you have to maintain the negative creation of you as YOU? Everything that is times a godzillion, will you destroy and uncreate all that? Right and wrong, good and bad, POD and POC, all nine, shorts, boys, and beyonds.

This is a powerful process. You may want to run this thirty times a day for thirty days. And here's another:

What repetitive patterns of negativity are you using to create your body? Everything that is times a godzillion, will you destroy and uncreate all that? Right and wrong, good and bad, POD and POC, all nine, shorts, boys, and beyonds.

Being the Master of Your Fate

Some people misidentify negativity as the source of who they are, and thus create it as a repetitive pattern—but the negativity isn't the source. It's YOU who are the source. You are the source beneath the negativity. You are the source for the creation of your body, your life, your living, and your money.

A couple of years ago, I watched a movie called Invictus, which is about Nelson Mandela, a truly great man who did not create himself from negativity. The title of the movie was taken from a poem by the English poet, William Ernest Henley. It's about being downtrodden and destroyed and still knowing that you're the master of your fate and the captain of your soul. This poem got Nelson Mandela through twenty-seven years of hard labor and confinement in a ten-foot by ten-foot jail cell. I highly recommend this movie, because it's about stepping up to the willingness to be great. It also shows how Mandela forgave the people who did him in. I think he was grateful to them for inspiring him to be the strength he truly was. Because of this experience, he was willing to look at the world from a totally different point of view.

If you were willing to look at the world from a totally different place and willing to be everything you are, how much would you change your body? How much would you change your finances? How much would you change your reality?

Everything that is times a godzillion, will you destroy and uncreate it all? Right and wrong, good and bad, POD and POC, all nine, shorts, boys, and beyonds.

"This Is a Disaster"

When something "ends," it is never the end. It is a transmutation into something that's going to be greater. When something goes in a direction you don't wish it to go, realize a door has opened to a new possibility. Don't move into a repetitively negative perspective like "this is a disaster" or "everything went up in smoke." That's the repetitive pattern of destruction of living. I learned long ago that whenever something seemed like a disaster, it was time to go out and celebrate—because it was a start of a whole new possibility.

A friend of mine got fired from her well-paying job. I said, "Come on, let's go out and celebrate!" She was so depressed she didn't want to celebrate, but I said, "You are going out to celebrate!" We went out, and I bought her a bottle of champagne and some pie. I said, "Here's to the beginning of a whole new life for you!"

> She said, "I never looked at it that way!"
>
> I said, "You didn't get fired. You just had an old door open up to a new possibility."

If you don't start living your life, you ain't going to have one. Right now is your 911 call. It's an emergency! Most people cry, "Emergency! Emergency!" and then they return to the repetitive pattern of "Wah, wah, wah! I need an ambulance!" Don't become the wha-ambulance. Get ambulatory. Get moving. Start creating your life. It's an emergency right now! If some living isn't done on this planet soon, this place is going to dry up and blow away. We've got to get some people to look at the world from a different place!

When you unlock your limitations around not owning your body and your money, you will start to trust yourself more. At some point, you and your body will start to be the magic you truly be. You will step into a whole new world. The things that you were doing and the things you were holding onto won't fit into the new life you're creating, so they will have to leave.

Getting It "Right"

Whenever you do a repetitive pattern, you're not making a choice and asking a question. Instead you're making a choice and trying to get it right, which is a judgment—and when you go into judgment, you are choosing not to perceive, know, be, and receive everything that's possible. Instead you try to figure out what's going on for other people, so you can get it right and fit into what they expect.

Addiction is one of the elements of repetitive patterns. People who do addiction have a tendency to repeat the same actions over and over again when they are in similar circumstances. They make choices that come out of the last circumstance they were in that was similar to their current situation, and they think that they're going to get a different result. Most of us do this. We tend to believe that we should do the same thing over and over again and eventually we're going to get it right. No! It is not about getting it right, it's about getting the awareness of what our choices are really going to create and knowing what we would like to create instead.

Tool: Choosing for Consciousness

There is a way not to loop back into old patterns. It's choosing for consciousness. You make a choice. You say:

- *Okay, I am making this choice and that opens the door to a certain number of potentials.*
- *Then you ask a question:*
  Where am I going from here? or
  What's next? or
  What else is possible?

When that question intersects with that potential, a new reality gets created.

What physical actualization of the terminal and eternal disease of the choice of the CCCRs for the creation of consistent, repetitive patterns of life and body do you have that maintains what you cannot change, choose, and institute as a totally different choice, possibility, and life? Everything that is times a godzillion, will you destroy and uncreate it all? Right and wrong, good and bad, POD and POC, all nine, shorts, boys, and beyonds.

If you want to create something different,
you have to do something different.

Tool: Ten-Second Increments

Living is about being in the ten-second increments of every moment so you are present for whatever occurs and capable of moving on to different things, if that's what you choose. It's about being in choice—not judgment. When you live in ten-second increments, you make every choice good for ten seconds. You choose something. Maybe your choice will turn out to be a stupid choice. What do you do then? You ask, "Well, what would I like to choose now?" You may say, "Okay, that's a better choice" or you may say, "That's not good enough." Then what do you do? You ask, "What else would I like to choose?"

You don't need to limit yourself to the results of your choice. You just choose again. If you chose to be with somebody in ten-second increments, how long would you stay with them? Ten seconds. And then what do you do? You choose again. Do you want to stay another ten-seconds? Most people think they're making their choices forever. In that first ten-seconds, they make a choice to be together—then they get married and live unhappily ever after.

I keep my life in ten-second increments as much as possible. I look for the joy and the adventure. Every day is a new thing. Ten seconds is a long time.

> Years ago a little boy showed up at our neighbor's house.
>
> He was seven years old. Our neighbor hadn't seen him before, and she asked him, "Where do you live?"
>
> He said, "Over there, about a mouse's mile."

He lived next door, but from his perspective, it was a mouse's mile. It turned out the little boy had leukemia, and he died very young. He often visited old people who were in the hospital, and he would say to them, "I'm dying, but it's not that bad. It's easy. Don't worry about it. You'll be fine when you die." He was trying to give them the awareness that it's okay to die. His point of view was "You have to be in this moment." He was living in ten-second increments.

Yesterday I found a young woman to ride my horse while I'm traveling. A friend who I ride with was stunned because I went boom-boom-boom-done! I didn't interview a million people and contemplate for days about who to choose.

> All I did was ask the horse, "Can this woman ride you? Do you want her to ride you?"
>
> My horse said, "Yes."
>
> "Okay, good. Done!" It was as simple as that.

That's living in ten-second increments. Could I change my mind tomorrow? Absolutely—because I'm not stuck with the choice I made. It works or it doesn't.

Just do this: You've got ten seconds to live the rest of your life. What do you choose? Okay, those ten seconds are up. You've got ten seconds to live the rest of your life. What do you choose? Good, those ten seconds are up. You've got ten seconds to live the rest of your life. What do you choose? Most people have two choices given to them—and they think they have to choose between those two things. The third choice is the one they really want, but they were never allowed to choose that one. When you live in ten-second increments of choice, you realize "Oh, I can choose again, again, and again." You have more than three choices available. You start to create your life from there. Or, you try to solidify your life into a consistent pattern or a point of view or a judgment that makes it "right." Living in ten-second increments is a totally different way to live.

It's a Choice You Have to Make

Do you put a limitation on the joy you can have? Are you willing to love life only to a certain point? If you get past that hump, do you freak out and go back to your limitations? This is a choice you make. You need to recognize what you are choosing. Are you going to choose to freak out every time you get close to total pleasure and total ease—or not? I know people who get to the point where they are about to make a lot of money and they destroy their possibilities every time. Why? They believe that to have that kind of pleasure with money would be wrong. Is that wrong? No, it's just a choice. You have to ask, **"How would I like to live my life?"**

What makes life worth living to you? What did you come up with? Fun? Joy? Peace and ease? Being creative? You want to live a life that has loving, joyful possibilities in it. All the things that make life worth living—are you living that?

Justifying Your Choices

Sometimes people say things such as, "I understand what you are saying about choosing, but I still allow other people's limitations or their points of view to stop me."

I reply, "You don't allow other people's points of view to stop you! You simply choose to stop you. You're the only one who can stop you."

Then they'll say something like, "Well, I'm stopping me from choosing that because...."

I step in at this point and say, "Stop when you get to the "because." Anything that comes after the because is your justification. You keep justifying why you choose something so you can make it solid and real, as if that's the only choice you have."

You have a point of view that this is the way life is. But life has no "this is the way it is." What if it isn't that way at all? You have locked "the way life is" into existence with the positional HEPADs you have chosen. That is not the truth. It can be different.

As long as you know "this is the way it is," you don't have to change and you don't have to choose. Everything that is times a godzillion, will you destroy and uncreate it all? Right and wrong, good and bad, POD and POC, all nine, shorts, boys, and beyonds.

Have you ever heard someone say, "Well, I've chosen this. Now I have to live with it"?

I reply, "Why do you have to live with it? There are other choices. What other choices do you have?"

They ask, "What do you mean?"

> I say, "You could throw it away, you could give it away, you could walk away."
>
> They say, "No, I could never do that."
>
> I ask, "Why not?"
>
> They say, "Because I put my money into it."
>
> I say, "That doesn't mean anything. Are you making money more important than living?"

Did you spend money on your education? If it wasn't right for you, did you walk away from it—or did you try to prove it was right that you should do all the things that you learned? Did you hate the career you chose so much that you didn't want to do it? Did you force yourself to do it anyway? Did you say, "Well, I've got to do it because I put all that money, time, and energy into learning how to do it. I've got to prove that it was the right choice"?

I watch people do this in relationships. They know the relationship is not working, but they do it anyway.

> I'll ask, "How long have you been married?"
>
> They'll say, "Twenty years—but it's not working."
>
> I'll ask, "Why don't you do something different?"
>
> They'll say, "No, I have to prove it works. I have to prove I made the right choice."

Nice, eh? What if you realized, after doing all of that, that it was stupid? Instead of forcing yourself to plow on, what if you simply asked, "What would I like to choose now?"

Choosing from the Kingdom of We

What if you made choices from the Kingdom of We? The Kingdom of We is about us, as the beings that we are, and what we wish to create. The real power of the Kingdom of We is being able to choose what works for us and everybody else. Choosing for you can be choosing for the Kingdom of We. You include all the other people in your life when you choose. You choose what works for you and for everybody else.

Most of us have learned that the only time we choose for ourselves is when we choose against somebody else. We think choosing against someone else is choosing for ourselves. It isn't. Choosing from the Kingdom of We gives you far more freedom than choosing against somebody else's point of view.

At one point, Dain got a new TV with all the bells and whistles. My daughter asked him if she and her friend could watch a movie on it while we were out of town.

> Dain said in stern voice, "Yes, but you better take care of it, young lady."
>
> I asked, "Dain, how were you treated when your parents got something new?"
>
> He said, "They used to say that kind of thing to me."
>
> I asked, "What if you treated others the way you *should* have been treated instead of the way you *were* treated? Were you always a responsible kid?"
>
> He said, "Yes, I always took care of everything."
>
> I asked, "Do you think my daughter is a responsible kid?"
>
> He said, "Yes, she is."

> I asked, "So why don't you treat her the way you should have been treated?"
>
> Dain called my daughter and said, "You can watch my TV any time you want," and instantaneously his world expanded.

My daughter's world hadn't contracted because of what he'd said—because she knows she's responsible. But his world had contracted when he tried to teach her a lesson based on the lesson his parents had been trying to teach him. That's not the way it needs to be! In order to create the world you'd like to have, you need to choose how you *should* have been treated, not how you *were* treated. It always expands you. That's the Kingdom of We—knowing what was done to you and knowing what could have been done for you, and choosing from that.

What would it take to generate an extraordinary life that works for you and your family?

Are You Trying to Find a Reason to Live?

Sometimes people tell me they are trying to find a reason to live. I ask, "What does the word *live* mean? What kind of word is *live*?" It's a verb. And what's a verb? It's an action. Are you living—are you really living—or are you busy looking for your life? Do you tell yourself a story about how you can't, how you won't, and how you shouldn't? Do you say to yourself, "Well, I ought to be able to—but I can't because ___"? Or is every ten seconds a joy for you? Is every ten seconds a new possibility?

What is stopping you? You.

What is stopping me? Me.

If you don't start living life, you ain't going to have one.

Chapter 12

Humans And Humanoids

You create yourself as a human when you actually are not. You're a humanoid.

But even to say that you are a humanoid is a limited point of view.

You're really an infinite being.

The truth is that you are an infinite being with an infinite body. You are energy, space, and consciousness—and you've created a molecular structure (your body) that you hold together so people can see you. You keep trying to create yourself as solid and "real" so you can be in agreement with everyone else in this reality—but that's not what you truly are. When you try to be like other people, you have to create the same pain, solidity, and limitations they have in their lives. To do this, you try to make yourself feel human—when what you actually are is a humanoid.

Humans are basically lead weight. Most of them are not energy, space, and consciousness. They like the heavy life. They believe that misery loves company, and they are miserable so they can have company and be just like everyone else. Would you be willing to let go of your "misery loves company" point of view and become so frigging light and airy that nobody wants to be around you? Would you be willing to be the humanoid you truly be?

The idea that no one will want to be around you is actually a lie. When you're light all the time, people love to be around you. In fact, nobody wants to go home. People come to our house and they say, "Oh, I just love hanging out with you. It feels so good here." They arrive at the door and say, "Hi, I just stopped by for a cup of tea." Four hours later as I walk them to the front door, I say, "It was so nice having you."

Humanoids Create the Great Possibilities

You may have seen people who live in a way you'd like to live. Their lives are about experiencing the elegance and aesthetics of life or enjoying the adventure of life or doing things that make the world a better place. Those people are humanoids. Humanoids are willing to have more, be more, and do more. They create all the great art, the great literature, the great possibilities, and the great ideas. That's you. How do I know that? Because you're reading this book!

Let's say you come up with a brilliant idea that will make people more money. You say, "Hey, I've got this great idea." The humans say, "Nope, you can't do that. We're not changing. We've always done things this way, and this is the way we'll always do them." Humans always have the point of view of

"No, you can't do that." When this happens, you may judge yourself as wrong. You aren't wrong—it's just that humans tend to judge others—and they like things to stay the same.

Humans Judge Everything—Except Themselves

Humans tell you how wrong you are and say things like, "If you would just do things the right way and stop spending all your money on the stupid stuff you're doing, you'd be fine. Sit down, have a beer, turn on the TV, and become a couch potato." Humans never judge themselves. They know they're right and you're wrong. It's just the way they function.

Humanoids are just the opposite. Humanoids judge themselves—but not other people. Your viewpoint is "I'm wrong, I'm terrible, I'm bad, I don't know what I'm doing, I should be better, I can't get anything right." You're always in judgment of yourself. You judge yourself relentlessly—despite all the great things you do. You even say, "I'm so judgmental." No, you're not judgmental; you're just aware. You're aware of other people's judgments of themselves or others—and you assume (because you are aware of them) that those are your judgments.

Humanoids at Work

Humanoids are often accused of working too fast or making other people look bad. If you're a humanoid, people tell you to slow down. You've had more jobs than anybody else you know. It's not that you *can't* keep a job; it's that you don't *want* to keep a job. The only jobs you have lost are the jobs you didn't want in the first place, which is every single solitary one of them. Humanoids always have the point of view of "What else can we do? This will be fun! Let's try this!" The only way you can find out what you want to do is by doing things until you know that you don't want to do them again.

As a humanoid, you are a master of all trades and a jack of none. You can learn any job in three days to three weeks, and then you're bored, so you try to change it. A humanoid cannot have a lifelong career, because they need at least five different things going on in their life at one time in order to be happy and to succeed. If you're a humanoid, you never get anything accomplished if you have less than five things happening at once. You've got to add things to your life, because when you have many things going on at all times, you will easily complete projects and everything will work with ease.

This is simply a humanoid trait. It's not a *wrongness.* It's not a *rightness.* It's just the way it works. You have to be willing to see this, or you'll make yourself wrong for the fact that you can't focus on one career. I've known many humanoids who hear this and say, "Yes, but I need to choose a career. Everybody says I need to focus on one thing." The truth is that if you concentrate on one thing, you'll get bored and be ready to move on within a year. You will quit whatever you're doing and go on to something else. Recognize this in yourself—and add things to your life. You think that if you make your life simpler, it will be easier. Nope, that's not the way it works for you. Add more to your life, and it will become simpler and easier.

How many positional HEPADs must you have to slow you down enough to live in this reality? A lot? A little or megatons beyond megatons? Everything that is times a godzillion, will you destroy and uncreate it all? Right and wrong, good and bad, POD and POC, all nine, shorts, boys, and beyonds.

Humanoids in Relationships

Having a relationship is hard for you as a humanoid. You have sex with somebody three times and then you say, "You know what? We need to change a lot or else we can't continue. That's just the way it is."

If you're a humanoid, when you get divorced, you are likely to give everything to the other person, leave all the furniture behind, and walk away with nothing except your suitcase. Humanoids know they can succeed, but the other person probably cannot. It's "Oh well, I can handle it; you can't. I'll take the kids because you can't handle them. I'll take the debts and the problems and the difficulties, and I'll leave you everything that makes your life easier. I must be at fault because I'm the humanoid, and I didn't figure out how to make our life work." This is not in your best interest. Cut it out! Get your share!

Your Personal Handicap System

There's another thing that humanoids do. They create a personal handicap system so they don't stand out from the crowd. In order to keep from being all the greatness you truly are as a humanoid, you develop a personal handicap. A handicap is a deficiency, disability, or disadvantage you take on to equalize your abilities with the abilities others have. You take on some sort of condition to level the playing field in the game of life. You want to give the other guy a chance to shine. You are like the hare in the story of the *Tortoise and the Hare*. You go really fast and then you have to lie down to rest because you're exhausted or you are too far ahead and you don't want to be seen as being too much of a winner. You then let the tortoise catch up and pass you. You use a handicap to make sure you are part of the human race.

It's as if somebody will be out to get you if you aren't handicapped. In Australia, they call this the "Tall Poppy Syndrome." If you stand out from the crowd, someone will cut you down so you'd rather be equal to everybody else. Are you using a personal handicap system to make you equal with everyone else—and still failing at the task of equalizing yourself?

One of your primary personal handicap systems is looking at your body through the judgments of others so you can maintain the symbiotic relationship as true. You think you have a symbiotic relationship with others that dictates that you are a human. This is not so!

Do You Only See Your Human Body?

Are you trying to prove that you're human when you're not? When you look in the mirror, do you only see the human body that you have? You don't see your humanoid body because your judgments of your human body are all you can take in.

The first time I traveled with Dain and Raymond, a young guy from Australia, Raymond would get up every morning in his T-shirt and boxer shorts, go into the bathroom and come out in small Aussie-style briefs. Dain would go into the bathroom wearing his T-shirt and boxers and come out in a fresh pair of boxers and a new T-shirt.

> One day I asked him, "Have you ever been in a locker room with other guys?"
>
> He said, "Yeah, why?"
>
> I said, "Because every morning you come out with a new T-shirt and a new set of boxers. I understand the boxers, but I don't get the T-shirt. What's the deal?"
>
> Dain said, "I have an ugly body."

I was taken aback because that's not what I saw. I asked him to go into the bathroom, take off his shirt, and tell me what he saw.

He did that, and he ripped his body to shreds. The judgment that came out of his mouth about his body was horrifying.

> I said, "Could you go back in there and look at your body through my eyes?"

He did. I could actually feel him stepping into my head to look at his body, which was pretty funny. He said, "*That's* what my body looks like?" After that he stopped wearing those T-shirts because he saw what his body actually looked like.

Most of us look in the mirror and see only the judgments we have of our body. We never see our body as it really is. We only see it as the judgments we've created.

Look at your body through somebody else's eyes—and not through yours, because yours lie with the judgment.

Any part of your body that you judge is a place you have assigned as your personal handicap system. It's what you do to make yourself like everyone else and keep yourself at the same level. Have you made the size, shape, or form of your body the source of your handicap? Do you judge the padding you have around your middle? That could be your personal handicap system. Are you using your skin's disease as a way of creating the handicap? Are you creating your skin color as a way of maintaining your handicap? Are you keeping your psychological profile in place as a way of maintaining your handicap? Every judgment you use against your body is a way of handicapping yourself so you do not become a generative, creative, institutive item for creation and facilitation of and on the Earth.

When I became willing to look at my humanoid body, I'd get up in the morning, check myself out in the mirror, and my body would look really good. Then I'd walk out of the room, get a judgment about my body, check the mirror again, and my body would look totally different. Now when I get up in the morning I always wonder what I'm going to look like, because I know every day is another source of change. When I look in the mirror, I don't expect my body to look the way it looked yesterday. I get up and I say, "I wonder what I look like today." It's about being in curiosity of how you're going to show up. I look at my body and say, "Wow, I'm looking pretty good!" Then I walk out of the room and I ask, "What would my body like to wear that would allow it to look like everything it really is?" That's different from asking, "What am I going to put on today that won't make me look as old and ugly as I think I am?"

> *What physical actualization of the terminal and eternal disease of the choice of the CCCRs for the creation of being human do you have that maintains and entrains savoring the judgments rather than living at peace with your body? Everything that is times a godzillion, will you destroy and uncreate it all? Right and wrong, good and bad, POD and POC, all nine, shorts, boys, and beyonds.*

Taking on Other People's Pain, Suffering, and Trauma

Do you have a personal handicap system that requires you to take on other people's pain, suffering, traumas, dramas, upsets, and intrigues? Do you get exhausted all the time and you don't know why? Are you handicapped by taking weight or fat out of other people? Are you adding weight to your body in an attempt to keep you equal with the density and the insanity of the other people on the planet? Have you been siphoning off others' violence or killing energy? Are you keeping someone from turning into a serial rapist? Are the toxins in your body, the anger, rage, fury, and hate that you've taken on from others, worse than the pollution on the planet? Have you taken on a personal handicap system as a way of trying to heal the Earth, save the planet, stop the killing, or to put an end to the destruction that's going on around us?

Do you see that by taking on the extra weight, extra pain, extra suffering, or whatever it is, that you're trying to make yourself equal to every other human on the planet? You can't prevent these things by taking them on as your handicap. Would you like to give up this job now? You can give up your personal handicap system for helping all people in pain. You can give up your willingness to suffer when others aren't. You can give up the idea that it makes you somehow nobler to suffer and that it's better to be excluded than to be generative enough to include others in your reality.

Would you please give up all your personal handicap systems? Everything that is for you, will you destroy and uncreate all that? Right and wrong, good and bad, POD and POC, all nine, shorts, boys, and beyonds.

Exercise: Put your attention on your body. Which part of your body is your personal handicap system?

Everything you've done to make that part of your body the source for your personal handicap, will you destroy and uncreate all that? Right and wrong, good and bad, POD and POC, all nine, shorts, boys, and beyonds.

Everywhere you've decided that it's more important to hold onto your personal handicap system than it is to be ahead of the game, will you destroy and uncreate all that? Right and wrong, good and bad, POD and POC, all nine, shorts, boys, and beyonds.

Are You Showing Up as the Radically Different Being You Truly Be?

> I got a call today from a lady who said, "You're always infinite, aren't you?"
>
> I said, "Yeah, why would you be anything else?"
>
> She said, "Every time I talk to you, no sooner are the words out of my mouth than I know you're going to say, 'That's B.S. Cut it out.' I know before I finish my sentence that it's going to be one of those things that you will slap me about."
>
> I said, "Yeah, because I'm not willing for you to be finite unless that's what you want more than anything else in your life."

People often think being an infinite being means being without a body. They think that you can only be infinite if you have no body. We've been caught up in a Catch-22. We are born with the awareness that we are a radically different being and then we exhaust ourselves with our personal handicap system to prove that we're not the radically different being we truly are.

Everywhere you've bought that your body is the personal handicap system that keeps you from being an infinite being, will you destroy and uncreate all that? Right and wrong, good and bad, POD and POC, all nine, shorts, boys, and beyonds.

The personal handicap system is everything that does not allow you to actually have a sense of peace with your body and the sense that you can let your body choose what it wants to be, what it wants to look like, and what it really is. What if you were willing to have an infinite body instead of a finite body?

How many personal handicap systems have you installed in your body to make sure you never show up as the radically different being you truly be? Everything that is times a godzillion, will you destroy and uncreate it all? Right and wrong, good and bad, POD and POC, all nine, shorts, boys, and beyonds.

I'm not willing for you to be finite unless that's
what you want
more than anything else in your life.

Chapter 13

CELEBRATING YOUR LIFE

Whatever we do here, let's enjoy the hell out of ourselves!

When I was a kid, I had an aunt who lived in Santa Barbara. She had an elegant home with Oriental rugs and beautiful, comfortable furniture. She listened to opera, drank out of crystal glasses, ate from fine china, and had sterling silver flatware as her everyday silverware. She bought delicious pastries and bread at bakeries and always had high-quality food to eat. I wanted to live like that! It wasn't about "We can't afford that. We can't have that." I said, "I'm going to have this kind of furniture. I'm going to live with this intensity of beauty."

My family was utilitarian. Everything was about the utility of things, not the beauty of them. The only beautiful things we had in our house came from my aunt. My mother polished them and put them on a shelf. Her point of view was that if anything was really good, you put it in a cabinet to keep it safe. You didn't use it. My point of view is "If it's beautiful, use it!" That was my aunt's point of view as well.

In our family, the furniture went into one location and it never moved again. It was arranged the same way for my entire life. At my aunt's every time we visited, the furniture was in a different position. She moved it around. I said, "Oh! I like being able to change things! That's something I want to do."

Life Should Be a Celebration

My point of view is that life should be a celebration. You should celebrate living. You created your body; why aren't you enjoying it? What if the purpose in life was to enjoy your body every moment of every day? Are you doing that?

Our ninety-five-year-old friend, Mary, lived with us near the end of her life, and one Christmas, we gave her a set of 600-count sheets.

> She opened her gift and said, "Oh, how lovely! I'll save these for a special occasion."
>
> I said, "Honey, I haven't been seeing anybody sneaking into your bedroom at night, so you better be using these every day, because everytime you wake up in the morning, it's a special occasion."
>
> People were horrified that I would say such a thing. I said, "I'm sorry, it's true."

You can't enjoy your body if you're not waking up. Waking up should be the most joyful thing you get to do each morning. "I woke up! How cool is that? It's foggy today! Cool, I get to wear my cold weather clothes. Oh, it's sunny today. I get to strip naked." It's "What do I get to do today?" not "What do I have to do?" **"What do I get to do today that would be fun and joyful and part of living the life I would like to have?"**

Aesthetics, Decadence, Hedonism, and Elegance

If you're going to celebrate your life, there are four qualities you need in your life: aesthetics, decadence, hedonism, and elegance. ***Aesthetics*** is the willingness to have the pleasure and the beauty of every moment. ***Decadence*** is the willingness to take whatever you want and leave the rest. There is no need to hold onto anything or everything. ***Hedonism*** is the recognition that pleasure is the joy of living. What if you do life because it's pleasurable, not because you have to? ***Elegance*** is the willingness to use the least amount of energy to get the greatest effect. It's like a woman in a gorgeous black velvet dress adorned with a single diamond brooch. To live, to really live, is to have the aesthetics, the elegance, the hedonism, and the decadence of life.

My Mini-Me Hearst Castle

A long time ago, I looked at my life and I said, "I'd like to live in Hearst Castle. Will they sell it to me? No. Could I afford the upkeep on it? No. So how can I have a Hearst Castle? I'll make my own mini-me Hearst Castle," and that's what I've done. That's the way I choose to live. I want to be able to have a great dinner party with beautiful things. I now have a sterling silver tray that came from Hearst Castle. It was one of twelve salvers that they had in the castle that went to the children of William Randolph Hearst.

A lady who was married to one of the Hearsts received it in her divorce and she sold it because she wanted to mess with her ex-husband. Now I have it. How lucky is that?

You have to look at how you want to live. I wanted to live with that kind of aesthetic. I wanted to live with that kind of decadent elegance. I wanted to live with that kind of pleasure and hedonism, and I have created just that. I have created my life around those concepts because that's what works for me.

How would you like to live your life? Are you one of those people who say, "I'm satisfied with the pathetic life I live; I'm satisfied with my middle-class existence"? Even though I have a mini-me Hearst Castle, I am not satisfied with that. I want more because I'm that obnoxious thing called a humanoid. Humanoids always want more; they're never satisfied with what they have. It's never enough. If you're a humanoid, you will always want more. You will never be satisfied with what you've got. And it's okay! That's just the way it is. If you're into horses, you'll want a better horse. Could I have a better horse? Could I have a bigger one? Could I have a prettier one? Could I have another one? Could I have ten more? Could I have twenty more? Could I have thirty more? Recognize that the joy of living is always seeking greater and seeking more.

Are You a Sensualist?

When I was a little kid, people would come to our house and they would put their coats on my parents' bed. I'd go in and rub my fingers through all the fur coats because they felt so good. I loved velvet because it felt so soft. I loved anything that was squishy, pretty, slick, or shiny. Do you like to feel things? If you do, you are a sensualist. You like to touch things, and you like being touched. If you will acknowledge that you are a sensualist, you can bring somebody into your life who will love touching your body because he or she is a sensualist as well. Being a sensualist is part of being a hedonist. Have you not acknowledged that you are a sensualist? Please do that.

Do you eat more than your body needs as though that's a form of sensuality and hedonism that you can actually own and have? It doesn't have to be that way; you could just feel your body parts. Do you ever caress your body in the way that you would like it to be caressed by others? You should—because your body likes that.

Clutter

Clutter is what many people use instead of living decadently. They think having too much stuff is abundance. That's not abundance. Abundance is the willingness to receive and have anything and everything and to choose what really works for you. Too much stuff is the substitute for true abundance. Don't substitute things for abundance.

I live with quality stuff; I go through my things and I give away or sell anything that doesn't meet my standards of today. Are you trying to create your life from yesterday? Would you like to give up creating your life from yesterday and start creating it from tomorrow?

> Someone recently told me, "I now have so much stuff that I live in clutter."
>
> I said, "When you have so much stuff that you are surrounded by clutter, you need to start asking, 'What wants to live with me? What here has enough quality for me to keep?' Get rid of the rest of it."

People look at the things they have cluttering up their life and they say, "Oh, this came from my family."

I say, "Yeah, and it's frigging ugly."

They know it's ugly too. They keep it in the closet and let it take up space because it came from the family. "It came from my family so I must love it." No, just because it came from your family doesn't mean you have to love it. It's ugly. That it came from your family means nothing.

Stop hoarding. That's not having—that's holding. ***Having*** is the ability to have anything and choose anything. ***Holding*** is latching onto a point of view or a thing as though it fulfills something. Things do not fulfill anything in your life. Retail therapy is not the source for living. You have to ask, **"Does this work for me? Do I need, want, require, or desire this?"**

You don't need to hold onto something because it came from the family. Give it to another family member. If there isn't a member of the family who wants it, sell it! Or give it away. If you don't totally love something, why are you living with it? You should live with what you love totally. Anything you don't love totally, get rid of it!

Years ago when I was in the antique business, I often met people who saved all kinds of stuff. They would say, "This was my grandmother's so it must be beautiful." No, the only reason it has been around for one hundred years is because it was so ugly that someone put it in a closet! Get rid of it! I wanted to start my own TV antique show called "Antique Roadkill," where I took really ugly, old stuff and said, "This should have died one hundred years ago!" Whack!

Life Is an Orgasm: Why Ain't You Having One?

I had a conversation recently with someone about what happens when she feels joy so intensely that she can't stand it. She said she felt like she needed to back away from it.

I asked, "Why do you say you can't stand it?"

She said, "It's almost like there is too much pleasure."

I replied, "You're rejecting the idea of having a life based on pleasure because you don't want the intensity of the pleasure."

She asked, "Well, what should I do when I perceive myself backing away or resisting the pleasure that's possible?"

I said, "Move into it. Force yourself to move into it. It's not 'Wow, how much champagne can I drink to get rid of this feeling?' It's 'Move into all the pleasure that's possible.' If you actually go into the pleasure, you may begin to vibrate with orgasmic possibility.

What you're doing now is looking for the pleasure in life as though there's something that will give you pleasure—and then, after that, it's over. This is why most people have sex. They're looking for the pleasure of life, which is, 'Okay, I had an orgasm. That's done.

Now what? Take a shower.'"

Most people can't have an ongoing intensity of pleasure with their bodies. What if you began to function from that kind of orgasmic energy all the time? What if you were willing to function as a complete hedonist whose whole purpose of life was to seek the pleasure of living?

If you are in the orgasmic quality of living, then everything is a pleasure that keeps expanding the possibility of greater pleasure. It's a different reality. You've got to be willing to step into that, but every time it comes up, you say, "No, that's too intense, I can't stand it. It's almost painful to be that happy." No, it's not. It's not painful at all. Do you mean there's a capacity for greater and greater orgasmic living? Yes, that's what I mean. But you've got to be willing to have the joy, decadence, aesthetics, elegance, and the hedonism of living.

What choice for not having the total joy, decadence, aesthetics, elegance, and hedonism of living can you now destroy, uncreate, and choose? Right and wrong, good and bad, POD and POC, all nine, shorts, boys, and beyonds.

Living is an active state of being present in
every moment and
enjoying the heck out of it no matter what occurs.

Chapter 14

The Target For Your Future

I would like to invite you to recognize your body as a gift—not a difficulty.

I would like you to recognize that you now have tools that will allow you to enjoy your life, your living, and your body. You can now create a future that will be an invitation to you to make your life as indefinite as it can possibly be.

I would like you to recognize that every moment of every day can gift you with the pleasure, joy, possibility, choice, and contribution of everything giving to you—and you giving to everything else—creating something greater than you ever thought possible.

Glossary

Be

In Access Consciousness, the word be is used to refer to you, the infinite being you truly be, as opposed to a contrived point of view about who you think you are.

Bars

The Bars are a hands-on Access process that involves a light touch upon the head of thirty-two contact points that correspond to different aspects of one's life. These points are called Bars because they run from one side of the head to the other.

Clearing Statement

The clearing statement is a tool you can use to change the energy of the points of view that have trapped you in unchanging situations. To use the clearing statement, ask a question designed to bring up the energy of what has you trapped, including all the crap built on it or hiding behind it, then say or read the clearing statement to clear the limitation and change it. The words that make up the clearing statement are:

> *Everything that is, times a godzillion, destroy and uncreate it all. Right and wrong, good and bad, POD and POC, all nine, shorts, boys, and beyonds.*

Right and wrong, good and bad is shorthand for: What's good, perfect, and correct about this? What's wrong, mean, vicious, terrible, bad , and awful about this? What's right and wrong, good and bad?

POC is the point of creation of the thoughts, feelings, and emotions immediately preceding whatever you decided.

POD is the point of destruction immediately preceding whatever you decided. It's like pulling the bottom card out of a house of cards. The whole thing then falls down. Sometimes, instead of saying "use the clearing statement," we say, "POD and POC it."

All nine stands for the nine layers of crap that we are taking out. You know that somewhere in those nine layers, there's got to be a pony because you couldn't put that much shit in one place without having a pony in there somewhere. It's shit that you're self-generating, which is the bad part.

Shorts is the short version of: What's meaningful about this? What's meaningless about this? What's the punishment for this? What's the reward for this?

Boys stands for nucleated spheres. Have you ever seen one of those kids' bubble pipes? You blow and you create a mass of bubbles. You pop one bubble and the other bubbles fill in the space. No matter how many bubbles you pop, you can never change it!

Beyonds are feelings or sensations you get that stop your heart, stop your breath, or stop your willingness to look at possibilities. It's like when your business is in the red and you get another final payment notice and you say Argh! You weren't expecting that right then.

Fealties and Comealties

A fealty is a sense of faithfulness and obligation to another person, group, or thing. Originally fealties were obligations of loyalty owed by a feudal vassal to his lord. Comealties are blood oaths.

Molecular De-Manifestation

When you want something to disappear or go away, you molecularly de-manifest it. In other words, you ask the molecules to change their structure so they become something else. You are actually changing the molecular structure of something so it ceases to exist. This works with things like tumors, arthritis, and calcium deposits—and apparently fat cells and toxins as well. They disintegrate and go away. You put your hands on the area you're addressing and say:

> *Molecularly de-manifest, right, wrong, good, bad, POD and POC, all nine, shorts, boys, and beyonds.*

Once you get it started, it will continue to run.

MTVSS (Molecular Terminal Valence Sloughing System)

MTVSS is a hands-on process to activate your body. It's the tool of choice for undoing almost any malfunction of the body. It can also have a major effect on the immune system, especially when it's done on the joints. It's also a system that you can activate when you're exercising.

MTVSS as a hands-on process is a great way to rev up your immune system and prevent colds and flu. You can do MTVSS on yourself, but it's much more dynamic if somebody else does it on you. You plus you equals two. You plus someone else equals about one hundred.

The third eye, thymus, spleen, liver, and kidneys are the primary sources for your immune system. If you put your hands on those six spots, it will turn your immune system on to a degree that's amazing.

To run MTVSS on someone, place one hand over the person's third eye and the other hand over the thymus. Then ask for:

> *MTVSS and all the rest, known and unknown. Right, wrong, good, bad, all nine, POC, POD, shorts, boys, and beyonds.*

MTVSS should turn on immediately, which means almost instantly you will feel an energy running through your hands. Some people feel major heat; others feel a vibration. For some it gets cold, for others it feels like an electrical discharge. It's actually all of those things. Each of us perceives things in the way we're willing to perceive.

Continue to hold your hands over the third eye and thymus until you feel the energy stop. It may feel hot for a while and then all of a sudden the heat will dissipate. Then repeat this process with one hand over the person's liver and the other hand over their spleen. Do it once again with your hands over the kidneys.

If MTVSS doesn't turn on immediately, repeat: *Right, wrong, good, bad, all nine, POC, POD, shorts, boys, and beyonds* continually until you feel the energy turn on.

After you do MTVSS a few times and you start to get the energy of what it is, you can put your hands on the body and simply say "MTVSS."

Bodies are designed to be generative. Unfortunately we get stuck in pain, and that creates degeneration instead of our generative capacity. When we free up the energy and allow this process to work, bodies becomes more generative and "miracles" can occur.

MTVSS is also a system that you can activate when you're walking, running, hiking, or doing your workout, so your body accesses all the energies it needs to be vibrant and vital in its energetic movement. As you are moving, just say:

MTVSS and all the rest. Right and wrong, good and bad, POD and POC, all nine, shorts, boys, and beyonds.

When I do MTVSS, I can walk up the steep hills of San Francisco without stopping and my body starts to have more energy, more oxygen, and more of everything else I need. I feel like I could keep on going forever.

Secret Agendas
Secret agendas are decisions we make or conclusions we reach that we are not aware of. They are all the points of view you had in any lifetime.

Verbal Processing
Verbal processing refers to Access Consciousness processes that use the clearing statement.

About the Author

Gary M. Douglas

20 years ago, Gary Douglas started to develop Access Consciousness® with the knowing that a different way of functioning in the world must be possible. His Purpose with Access is to create a world of consciousness and oneness-where consciousness includes everything and judges nothing.

Simple, effective, and to the point, Access is a set of tools, processes and questions that enable people to create change in any area of their life.

Born in the American Midwest and raised in San Diego, California, Mr. Douglas has always been on a spiritual path, seeking deeper answers to life's mysteries. His innate curiosity has allowed him to question what didn't seem to be working in life and to seek alternatives to the popular views and accepted wisdom of today. He has been married twice and has four children.

Today, Mr. Douglas' workshops can be found in 25 countries and are offered by over 600 facilitators worldwide. Mr. Douglas continues to travel all over the world facilitating advanced classes on subjects ranging from bodies, the Earth, animals, conscious children, possibilities, relationships and money.

The techniques of Access Consciousness are being used worldwide to transform lives and bodies in private practices as well as in conjunction with addiction recovery, weight loss, business and money, animal health and many holistic health modalities, such as acupuncture and chiropractic care.

Mr. Douglas has written several books on the subjects of money, sex, relationship, magic and animals. In 2010, "The Place" became a Barnes and Noble bestseller.

To find out more, please visit:
www.GaryMDouglas.com
www.accessconsciousness.com
www.isnowthetime.com

Access Consciousness Core Classes

Access Consciousness™ classes provide verbal processing and simple tools for change that allow as much or as little change as you are willing to choose! What if you didn't require someone else to give you an answer... just some questions that could allow you to know what you know? Would that create greater possibilities for your life?

Access Consciousness™ offers eight Core Classes and many specialty classes which are all designed to give you greater ease, joy, abundance, choice and possibilities in your life. Many of the Core Classes have prerequisites that allow participants to move through into the advanced classes very quickly, if desired.

A comprehensive manual is provided in the Bars class through the Level 3 classes, containing detailed explanations, processes and tools discussed in class by the class facilitators. You will expand your awareness of what change is possible for you by asking questions of your facilitator. The advanced classes are free-form and class recordings enable you to go to deeper levels of change each time you listen!

Kids aged 15 and under come for free to all classes around the world. Ages 16, 17 and 18 pay half price. Everyone is included in Access Consciousness and your presence is considered a contribution to a greater possibility for the world.

The Core Classes listed below can expand your capacity for consciousness so that you have greater awareness about you, your life, this reality and beyond! With greater awareness, you can begin generating the life you always knew was possible and haven't yet created. What else is possible?

"Consciousness includes everything and judges nothing."
~ Gary Douglas, Founder, Access Consciousness.

Access Consciousness is a set of tools and techniques that are designed to give you the tools to help you change whatever isn't working in your life, so that you can have a different life and a different reality. Access Consciousness is a constantly evolving, changing, and altering the universe. It does not work from your cognitive mind. If your logical mind actually could create the results of change and difference that you would like to have, you would already be there!

Are you ready to explore the infinite possibilities?

For more information, please visit:
www.accessconsciousness.com

Access Bars

Do you remember the last moment in your life when you were totally relaxed, nurtured and cared for? Or has it been a little too long since you received healing and kindness without any judgment for your body or your being?

The first class in Access is The Bars. Did you know there are 32 points on your head which, when gently touched, effortlessly and easily release anything that doesn't allow you to receive? These points contain all the thoughts, ideas, beliefs, emotions, and considerations that you have stored in any lifetime. This is an opportunity for you to let go of everything!

Each Bars session can release 5-10 thousand years of limitations in the area of your life that corresponds with the specific Bar being touched. This is an incredibly nurturing and relaxing process, undoing limitation in all the aspects of your life that you are willing to change!

How much of your life do you spend doing rather than receiving? Have you noticed that your life is not yet what you would like it to be? You could have everything you desire (and then some!) if you are willing to receive lots more and maybe do a little less! Receiving or learning The Bars will allow this and so much more to show up for you!

The Bars has assisted thousands of people change many aspects of their body and their life including sleep, health and weight, money, sex and relationships, anxiety, stress and so much more! At the worst you will feel like you have just had the best massage of your life. At the best your whole life can change into something greater with total ease.

Taking The Bars class is a prerequisite for all Access Consciousness Core Classes as it allows your body to process and receive the changes you are choosing with ease.

Duration: 1 day
Pre-requisites: none

Foundation & Level 1

Have you noticed that this reality doesn't always work for you? Are you looking for the keys that will unlock the limitations of this reality and allow you to step into infinite possibilities? What if you could have everything you truly desire in life?

Access Consciousness is a pragmatic system for functioning beyond the limitations of a world that doesn't work for you. By looking at life's issues from a completely different perspective, it becomes easier to change anything. For anything to limit you, you must be functioning from some form of anti-consciousness or unconsciousness. So what can you choose instead?

Access Foundation is about getting out of the matrix of this reality. You will begin to uncover the points of view that are limiting you that if you were to change them would allow the possibility of functioning from question, choice, possibility, and contribution.

In Level 1 you will discover how to truly create your life as you desire it. This class will give you even greater awareness of you as an infinite being and the infinite choices that you have available. You will be excited by the possibilities of the quest "What Else is Possible?"

These two classes may be taken together or separately by Certified Access Consciousness Facilitators. You will get practical, real life tools including some hands-on body processes. The greatest potency is the ability to change and transform anything and everything.

Duration: 2 days per class
Pre-requisites: Access Bars (and Foundation to do Level 1)

Levels 2 & 3

These two classes are offered by Access Consciousness founder, Gary Douglas or Dr. Dain Heer. During these four days you will gain access to a space where you begin to recognize your capacities as an infinite being.

As you begin to recognize how different you are, you start becoming aware of the choices that you make, the choices you would like to make, and what you would like to generate as your life with ease...financially, in relationships, in your work and beyond....

Generating your life is different from creating it. For creation to occur, there always has to be destruction. Generating your life is a moment-by-moment increase in what else is possible. When you stop creating from your past you can start generating a future that is unlimited. What if sensing the possibilities could replace judgment of everywhere you are right or wrong?

What else would you like to add to your life? And what catalyst for change could you be in the world if you unleashed the real you? Would you be willing to function from the energy, space and consciousness you truly be? And would you be willing to be more of you than you have ever been before with ease, joy and glory? And maybe just a little bit of happiness too?

Duration: 4 days (2 days for Level 2 & 2 days for Level 3)
Pre-requisites: Access Bars, Foundation, Level 1

Access Body Class

What if your body was a compass or guide to the secrets, mysteries and magic of life?

The Access Body Class was created by Gary Douglas and Dr Dain Heer. Facilitated by Certified Body Class Facilitators, during these three days you will receive and gift numerous hands-on body processes that unlock the tension, resistance, and dis-ease of the body by shifting energy dynamically. There are over 40 hands-on processes, as well as lots of verbal processes in the Body Class manual that will allow you to deal with most issues that exist in bodies today.

People who have attended the Access Body Class have reported dramatic shifts and changes with body size/shape, overall relief from chronic and acute pain, and their relationships and money issues seem to get easier, too.

The Access Body Class is designed to open up a dialogue and create a communion with your body that allows you to enjoy your body instead of abusing it and fighting against it. When you start to change the way you relate to your body, you start to change how you relate to everything in your life.

Do you have a talent and ability to work with bodies that you haven't yet unlocked? What do you know? Are you a body worker—massage therapist, chiropractor, medical doctor or nurse—looking for a way to enhance the healing you can do for your clients? Come play with us and begin to explore how to communicate and relate to bodies, including yours, in many new ways.

Duration: 3 days
Pre-requisites: Access Bars, Foundation, Level 1

Energetic Synthesis of Being with Dr. Dain Heer

This class is unlike anything else on the planet! In this signature class, Dr. Dain Heer invites you and everyone else present to know what you know and to start contributing to the true possibility of change, expansion and consciousness for yourself, everyone around you and the planet.

> *"There has not been anything that produces this kind of change...the capacity to have a bigger and better life than I ever imagined...it is about having more of you."*
> *~Marilyn*

The Energetic Synthesis of Being is a unique way of working with energy, groups of people and their bodies simultaneously, created and facilitated by Dain.

During this 3-day intensive, Dain works simultaneously with the beings and bodies in the class to create a space that allows the change you are asking for to come into being. In working with one, the whole class is invited to that difference.

The result is an acoustical wave that invites a sense of peace and space that encompasses the class and contributes to a more conscious life and a more conscious planet. By choosing these classes, you are opening doors: doors to change, to awareness, and to a universe of oneness and consciousness.

You begin to be and receive energies you always knew were available but didn't have access to before. You'll discover that you no longer have to hide you, divorce you, go against what works for you and what you know is true for you.

By being these energies, by being you, you change everything; the planet, your life and everyone you come into contact with. What else is possible then? Would you be willing to come on the adventure and find out what that looks like for you?

Duration: 3 days

What is Energetic Synthesis of Being?

"It's a gift; an absolute gift."
"The connection to my body, with everyone and my life has changed"
"I know what it's like to be me...and it's pretty cool."
"I watched my whole world expand."
"It's kind of indescribable."

Being You, Changing the World Class

Do You KNOW there is something more? What if that "something" is YOU? What if you, being you, are all it takes to change EVERYTHING—your life, everyone around you and the world?

There is only one thing you are born to do. You were born to be...YOU!

Not the 'you' your partner, society or your parents want you to be. It isn't about being successful or DOING anything better. It is about BEING you! The energy you be.

Building on the tools delivered in Dr. Dain Heer's book **Being You, Changing the World**, this class presents the possibility of implementing deeply penetrating tools to effect profound change in your life. It's easy to do—all that is required of you is a willingness to ask for and choose to be the truth of you.

Fundamentally, it asks the questions: If you were being you-who would you be? Would you be willing to know what's really true for you? This is a class for the seekers out there. Always asking for more, being more, and looking for that "something" we all know is possible.

This is a unique 2.5-day class featuring a method Dain has developed and continues to expand. Together with the group, you'll explore the very energies of living. You'll get tangible, practical and transformative tools that will allow you to start finding out what is true for you and access your knowing of who you truly BE.

Throughout the days of this intensive, you'll receive an experience of being you that is impossible to describe and that you won't find anywhere else. What if you, being you, are the gift and change the world requires?

> *"This class was beyond anything I could ever imagine! I did not even want to go at first...I was so fed up with all those questions that are supposed to change things but that in my mind did not work at all. Now I am connected to the universal flow and aware of how quickly things change if I ask for them." ~Sonja*

Together with the group, you'll explore the very energies of living. You'll get tangible, practical and transformative tools that will allow you to start finding out what is true for you and access your knowing of who you truly BE.

During this class, you'll start to receive an experience of being you that is impossible to describe and that you won't find anywhere else. What if you, being you, are the gift and change the world requires? Is now the time?

Duration: 2.5 days

What people say?

I have spent a great deal of my life feeling very uncomfortable about myself, very unsure of myself and making myself wrong at every available opportunity. This class is an environment where it is not only OK to Be you, but where it is all about Being you, embracing you and coming out of that place of judgment and wrongness you have of you. It is a gift that is so wonderfully joyous, I can only hope that you can sense that space through these words—really.

The biggest thing I've noticed so far and that I've gotten about me after this class, is actually how much I really love life & living! How happy I truly am! How light I truly am! How much energy & exuberance I actually have! And here I was thinking that I didn't actually like living that much—not true!!

I look about ten years younger than I did last week and I've been jumping around like a mexican jumping bean wondering what's possible now with all this energy I have! How does it get any better than that?! This is what it is to BE ME........and I like it........a whole lot!!
~Naomi

Other Books

BY
GARY M. DOUGLAS & DR. DAIN HEER

The Place
By Gary M. Douglas
2010 Barnes and Noble #1 Best Selling Novel. "In this book you may find out what you have always been looking for, and how and where it may exist."

Divorceless Relationships
By Gary M. Douglas
A Divorceless Relationship is one where you don't have to divorce any part of you in order to be in a relationship with someone else. It is a place where everyone and everything you are in a relationship with can become greater as a result.

Magic. You Are It. Be It.
By Gary M. Douglas & Dr. Dain Heer
Magic is about the fun of having the things you desire. The real magic is the ability to have the joy that life can be.

Money Isn't the Problem, You Are
By Gary M. Douglas & Dr. Dain Heer
Offering out-of-the-box concepts with money. It's not about money. It never is. It's about what you're willingness to receive.

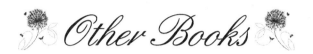

Sex is Not a Four Letter Word but Relationship Often Times Is
By Gary M. Douglas & Dr. Dain Heer
Funny, frank and delightfully irreverent, this book offers readers an entirely fresh view of how to create greater intimacy and exceptional sex.

Right Riches for You!
By Gary M. Douglas & Dr. Dain Heer
What if money could work for you instead of you working for money? This book offers tools to empower you to change your financial situation with ease and permanence. *As seen on Lifetime Television's Balancing Act Show.*

CPSIA information can be obtained
at www.ICGtesting.com
Printed in the USA
FSOW04n0259230316
18167FS

9 781939 261199